HEALTHY HABITS
WITH OR WITHOUT DIABETES
ACTIVITY BOOK

written by
FLOYD STOKES

illustrated by
SHEENA HISIRO

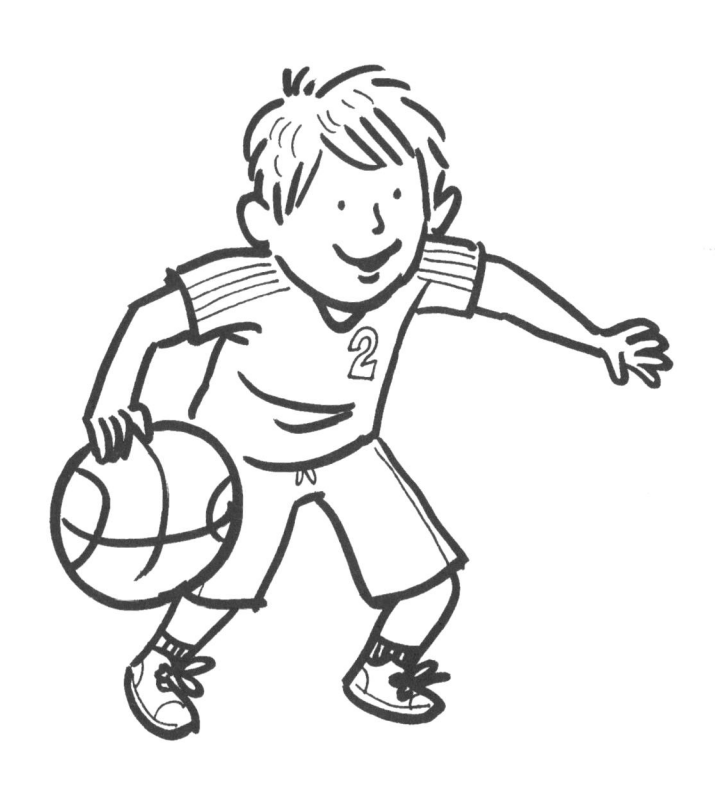

No part of this publication may be reproduced in whole or part, or stored on a retrieving system, or transmitted in any form or by any means, electronic, mechanical, photocopying, recording, or otherwise, without written permission of the publisher. For more information regarding permission, visit www.superreader.org.

A publication of the American Literacy Corporation for Young Readers

Text copyright © 2012 by Floyd Stokes.
Illustrations copyright © 2013-2014 by Sheena Hisiro.
Graphic Design by Sheena Hisiro.
First Edition, 2014. All rights reserved.

ISBN 978-0-9797871-9-5

PRINTED IN CHINA

Dear Readers,

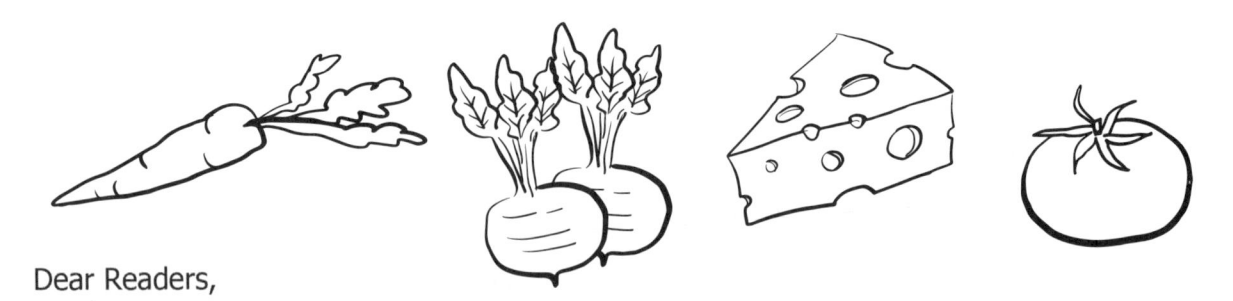

40 years ago when I was diagnosed with Type I (juvenile onset) diabetes my life expectancy with the disease was only 20 years. But thanks to the great advances in medicine and treatment, I live a busy and active life. I was also taught to eat a healthy diet, participate in moderate activity and manage my blood sugars, even at a very young age.

I realize that good nutrition and daily activity make me feel better, have more energy, and not be sick. You too can manage your health by making the best choices for your well-being.

This *Healthy Habits Activity Book* is chalked full of fun and educational activities. Great care has been taken to ensure that there are a variety of activities for children of all ages and levels. The book gives tips on how to stay active and make healthy eating a part of your daily life.

I am proud to be a part of the *Healthy Habits Activity Book* which was created in partnership with Capital BlueCross and the PinnacleHealth Auxiliary. My special thanks to Floyd Stokes, Sheena Hisiro, Joan P. Line, Barbara Terry, Phyllis Hicks, and all the people who helped to develop the book. Please enjoy.

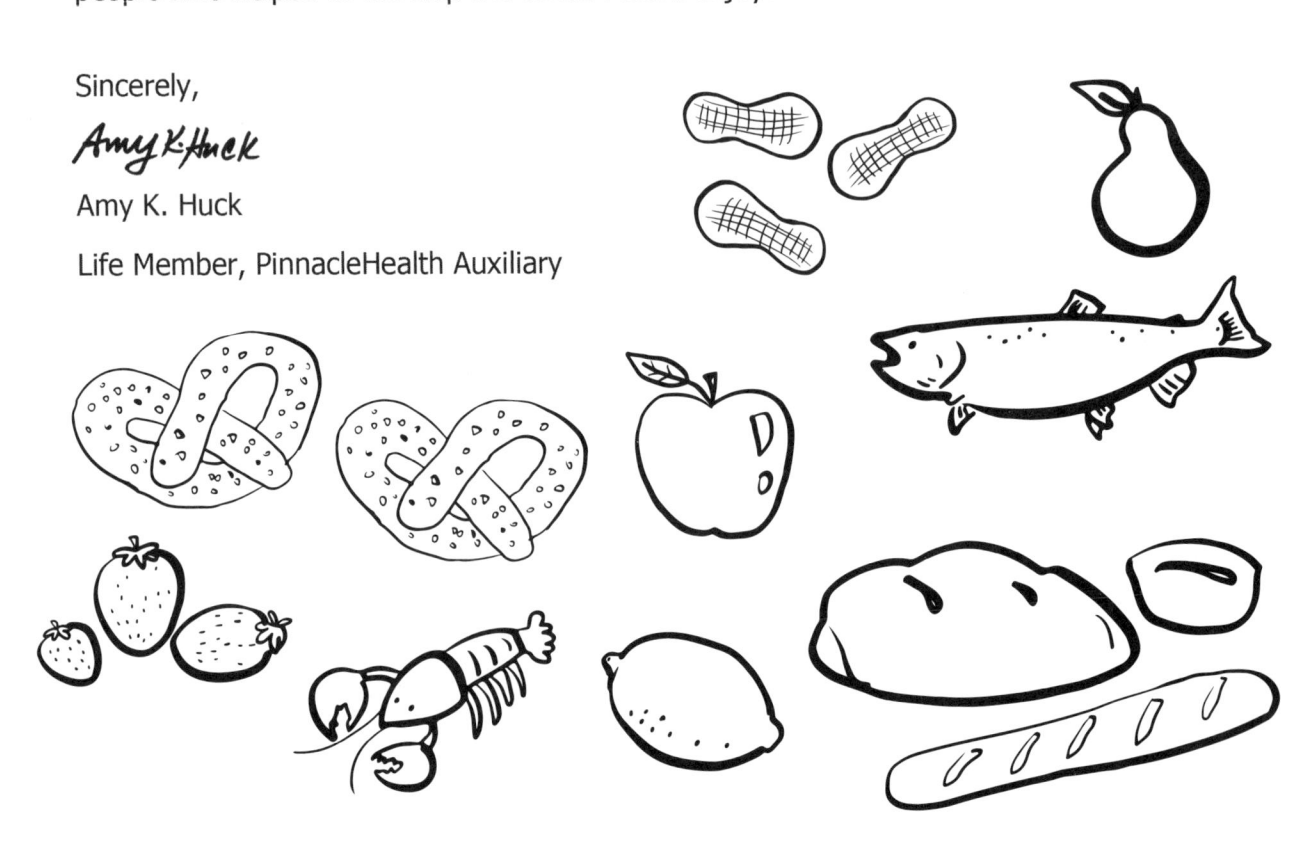

Sincerely,

Amy K. Huck

Amy K. Huck

Life Member, PinnacleHealth Auxiliary

MyPlate

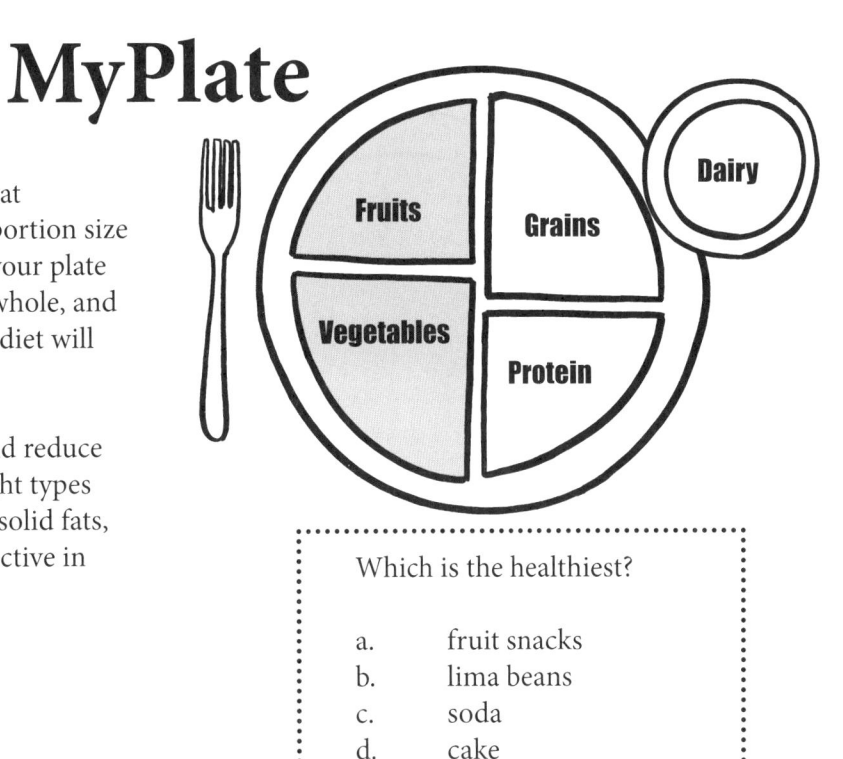

MyPlate helps you build a healthy plate at mealtime, and shows the recommended portion size for each different food group. Make half your plate vegetables and fruits, half of your grains whole, and your proteins small and lean. A balanced diet will also include Dairy, Fats and Oils.

Would you do something to feel better and reduce your risk for disease? You can! Eat the right types and amounts of food, limit foods high in solid fats, added sugars and salt, and be physically active in your own way.

Which is the healthiest?

a. fruit snacks
b. lima beans
c. soda
d. cake

Fruits and vegetables come from farms around the world, although most of us get them from the grocery store. Match each word or picture with the correct food group.

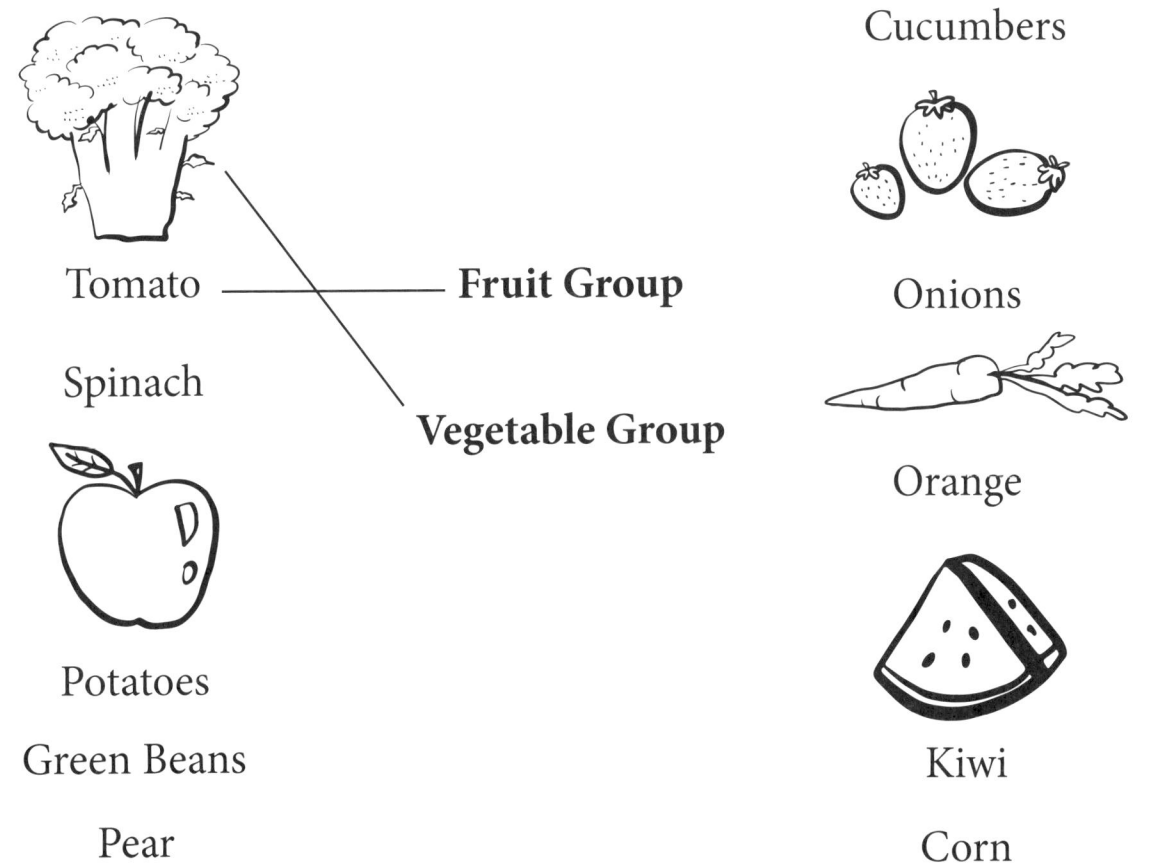

Tomato —— **Fruit Group**

Spinach

Potatoes

Green Beans

Pear

Cucumbers

Onions

Orange

Kiwi

Corn

Vegetable Group

Answer: b

Healthy Habits text by Floyd Stokes. Illustrations © Sheena Hisiro.

MyPlate

Draw a meal that has your favorite foods from all the food groups on the plate.

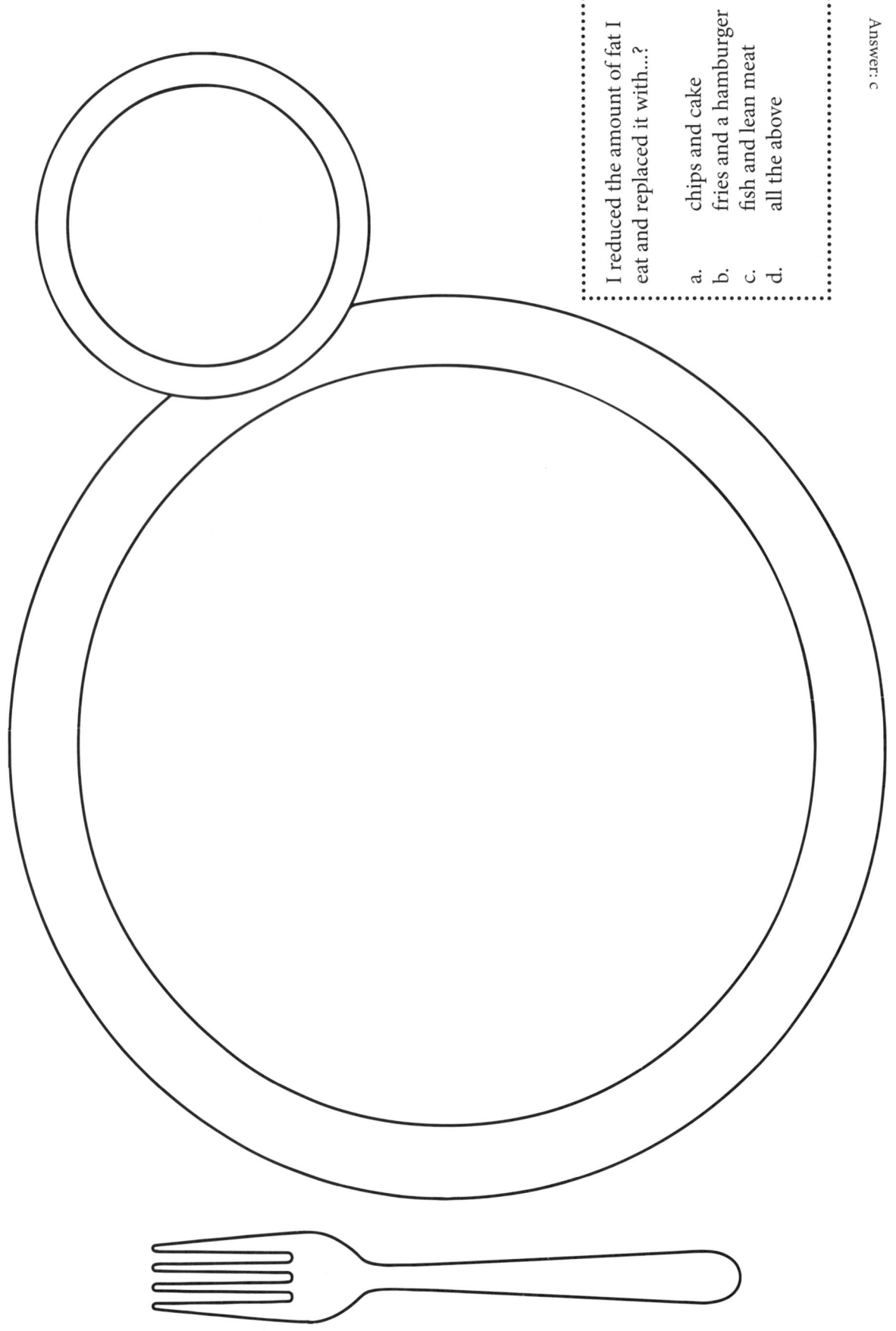

I reduced the amount of fat I eat and replaced it with...?

a. chips and cake
b. fries and a hamburger
c. fish and lean meat
d. all the above

Answer: c

Healthy Habits text by Floyd Stokes. Illustrations © Sheena Hisiro.

Stay Healthy Word Find

```
Y E S H X D I K A G P Q Q G K S F I T W
H S T K X M N C D N C Q N Q R G C U R E
W R Z J G I A E W C I O B A K E D N X W
G A E S R R M N R D R O I L C S C A A R
A X T D A D I O A T X D X L E T L H F P
X L N E U U T L S G E K H N J E I P F L
K Q Z A R C P X L M E X O Z R A N V T D
P D A N O Y E G A E D B D I A B E T E S
P X D D H Z N E M F D H O Q D P J C K U
Q T R O A S T E D U I N E E V L N J A Z
D I S E A S E W X Z S G E A N A X F H Q
J E F X G S B Y V R U C A A L E A N I U
V G I G D L A J M C C U L A C T E J O B
O Q E G M J O O L U I P B E Y C H G V M
Q D A O J T B C S R B C N Z S Q W Y K M
```

ACTIVE
BAKED
BALANCED
BONES
CURE
DIABETES
DISEASE
DOCTOR
DRINK
FIT
GRILLED
HEALTHY
LEAN
MANAGE
MUSCLES
PLAN
REDUCE
RELAX
ROASTED
STEAMED
STRONG
SUCCEED
WATER

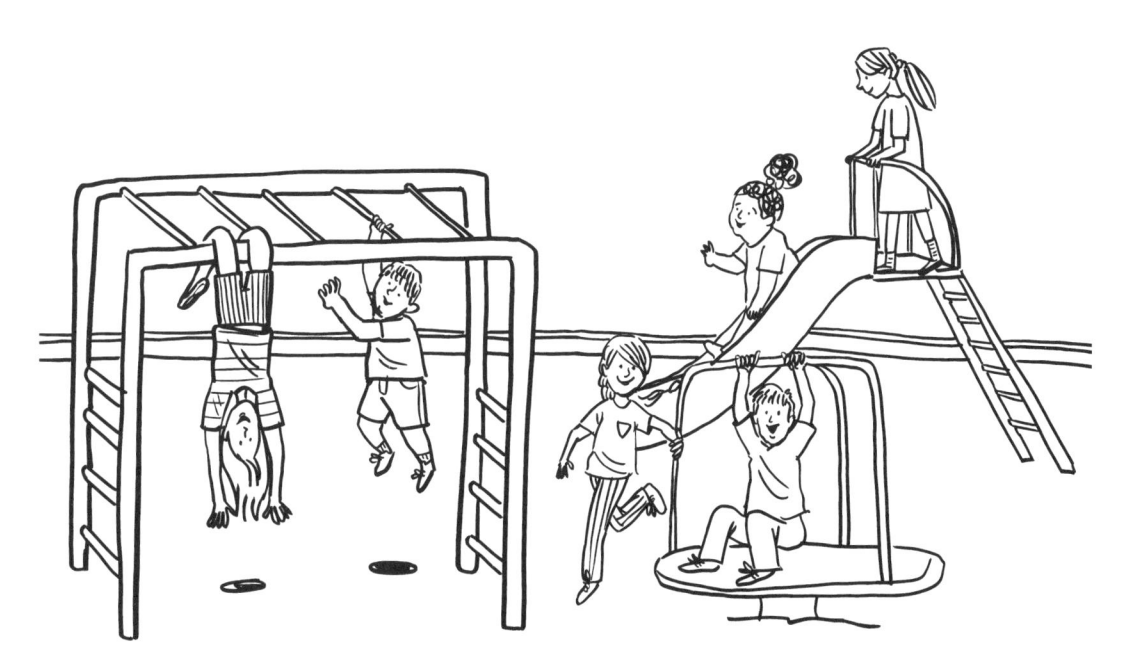

Healthy Habits text by Floyd Stokes. Illustrations © Sheena Hisiro.

Match a word on the left with a word on the right to complete a food name.

Skim _____	Rice
Frozen _____	Peppers
Ice _____	Burgers
Brown _____	Potatoes
Collard _____	Seeds
Chicken _____	Butter
Pinto _____	Milk
Veggie _____	Flakes
Peanut _____	Yogurt
Sunflower _____	Eggs
Red _____	Cream
Sweet _____	Beans
Corn _____	Greens

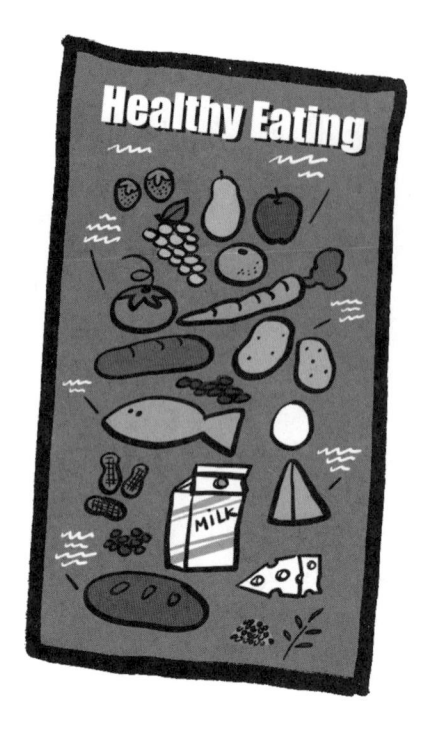

CRYPTOGRAM

A	B	C	D	E	F	G	H	I	J	K	L	M	N	O	P	Q	R	S	T	U	V	W	X	Y	Z
15	7	11	4	17	10	3	14	12	13	23	9	6	20	25	18	16	21	19	8	26	2	5	22	1	24

__ __ __ __ __ , __ __ __ __ __ __ __ __ __ , __ __ __ __
12 10 1 25 26   4 25 20 8   10 17 17 9   3 25 25 4

__ __ __ __ __ __ __ __ __ __ __ .
8 17 9 9   15 20   15 4 26 9 8

Who should help you develop a plan to manage diabetes?

a. Registered Dietitian
b. Nutritionist
c. Diabetes Educator
d. all of the above

Food Names
Skim Milk
Frozen Yogurt
Ice Cream
Brown Rice
Collard Greens
Chicken Eggs
Pinto Beans
Veggie Burgers
Peanut Butter
Sunflower Seeds
Red Peppers
Sweet Potatoes
Corn Flakes

Cryptogram
IF YOU DON'T FEEL GOOD,
TELL AN ADULT.

Answer: d

Healthy Habits text by Floyd Stokes. Illustrations © Sheena Hisiro.

Nuts About Nuts

FUNNY CORNER

What did the performing walnut say to the pecan?

Almond next

Which nut has beautiful eyes?

A Hazelnut

Diabetes affects...?

a. only adults
b. only men
c. only children
d. adults and children

ACORN
ALMOND
BEECH
BUTTERNUT
CASHEW
CHESTNUTS
HAZELNUT
HICKORY
PECAN
MACADAMIA
PISTACHIO
WALNUT

Choose unsalted nuts or seeds as a snack, or on food to replace meat or poultry. Nuts and seeds are a natural source of protein with a concentrated source of calories. So eat small portions to keep calories in check.

Answer: d

Healthy Habits text by Floyd Stokes. Illustrations © Sheena Hisiro.

Circle the item in each row that doesn't belong.

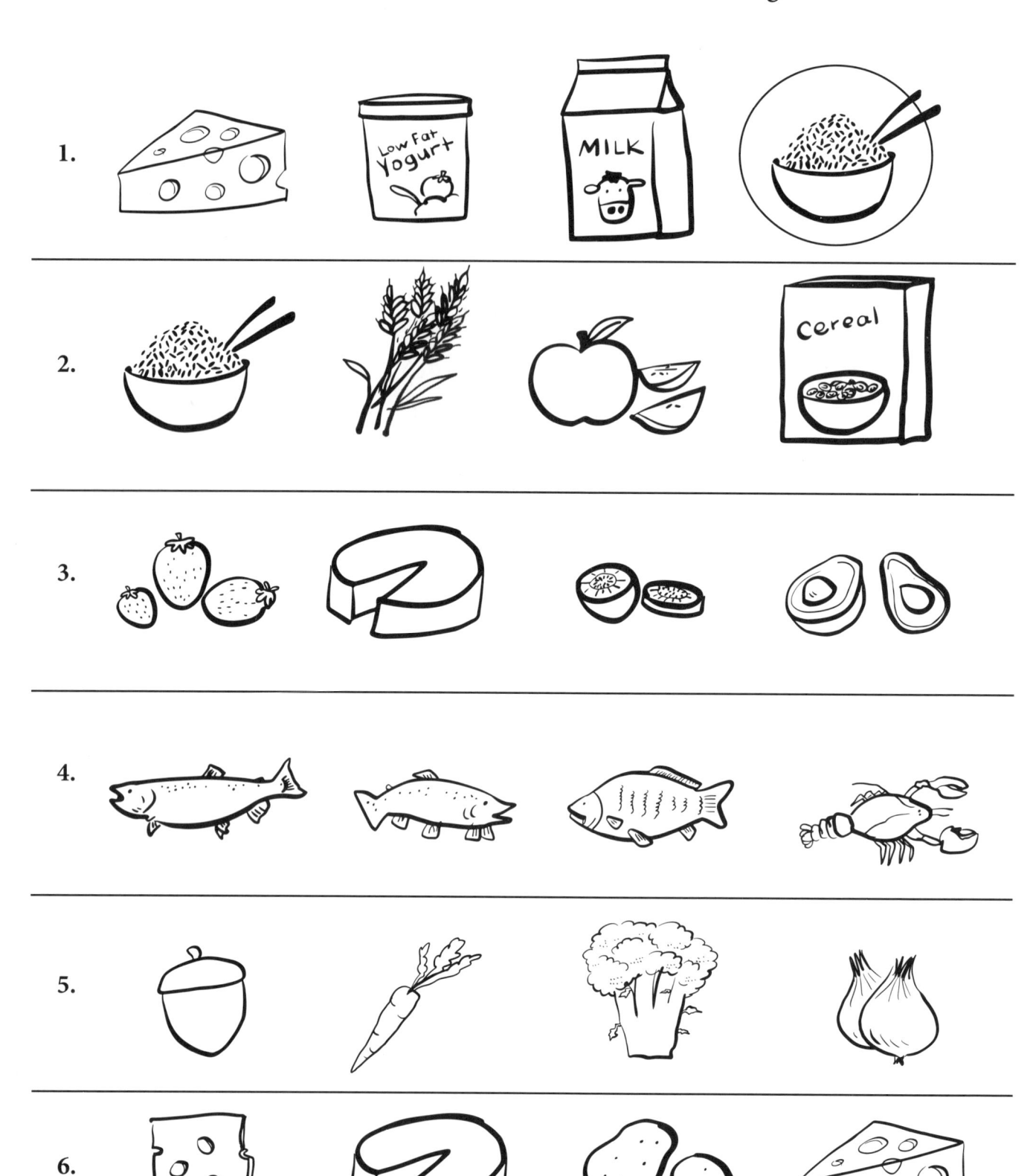

1.
2.
3.
4.
5.
6.

Healthy Habits text by Floyd Stokes. Illustrations © Sheena Hisiro.

Spot the Difference

There are 6 differences between these two pictures. Can you spot them?

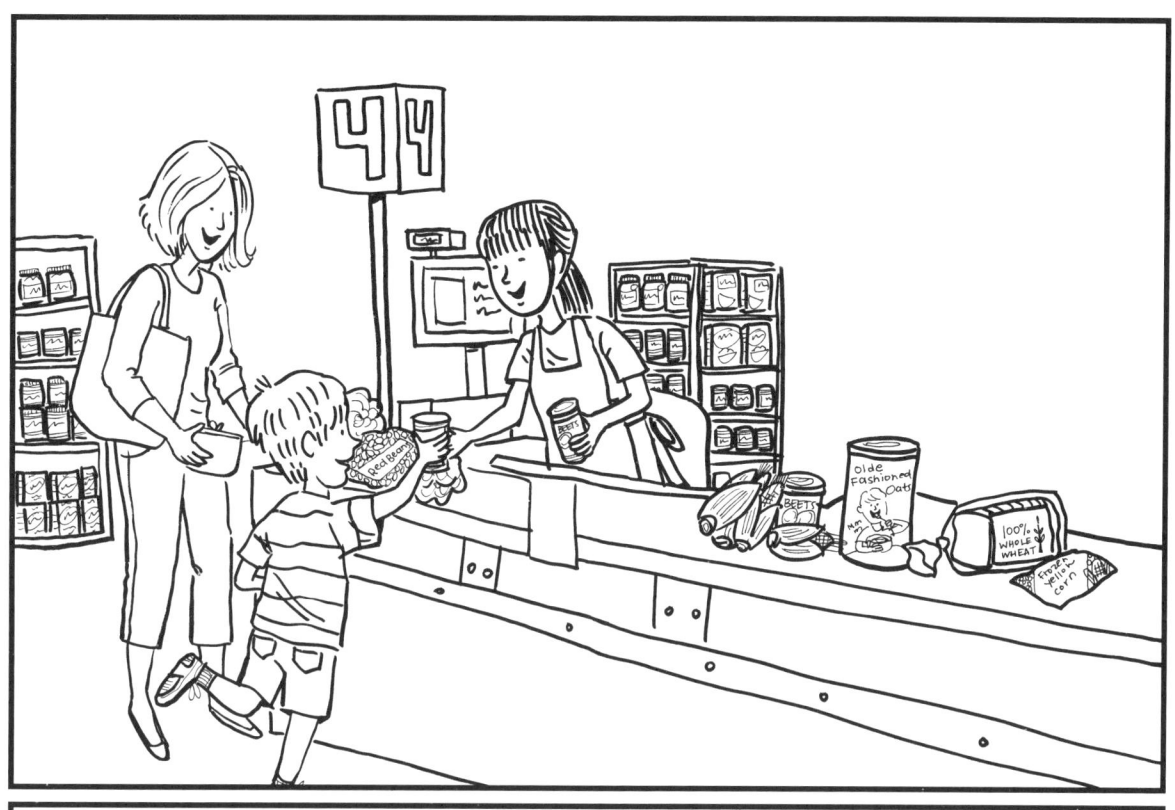

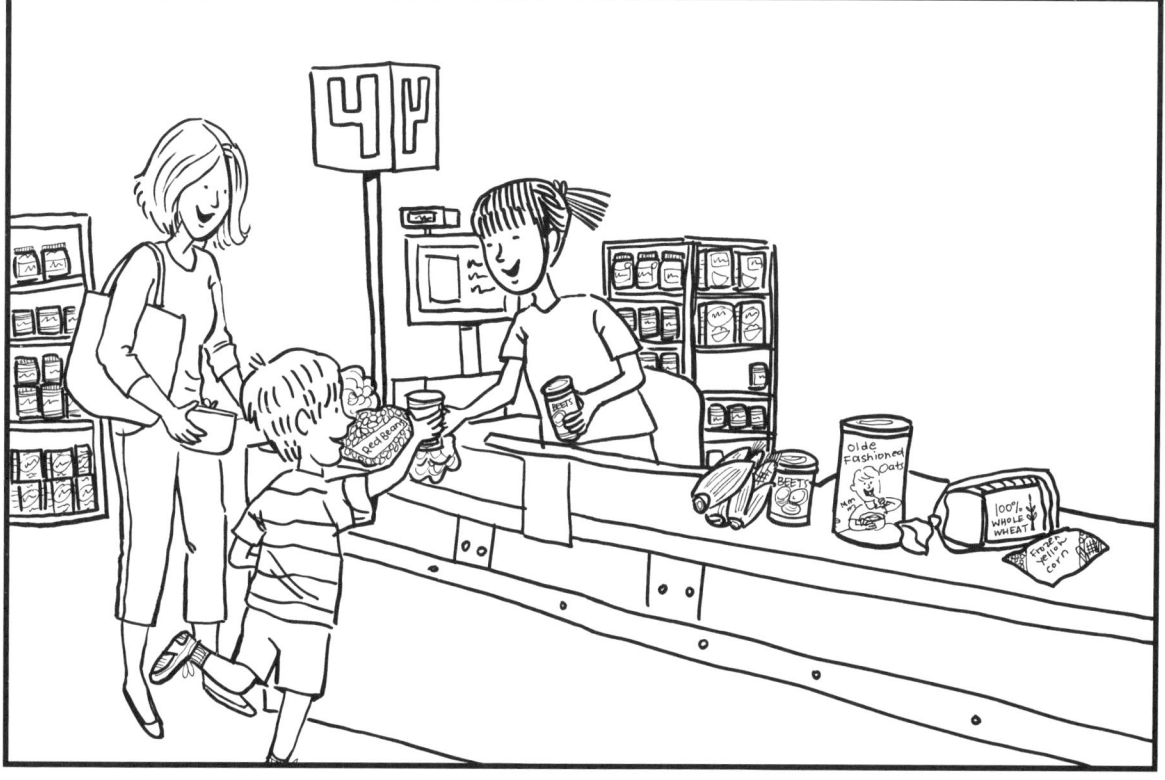

Healthy Habits text by Floyd Stokes.   Illustrations © Sheena Hisiro.

Word Scramble

CCLORBIO ☐☐☐☐☐☐☐☐
            8

LEUCETT ☐☐☐☐☐☐☐
          4

PCAIHNS ☐☐☐☐☐☐☐
        11   1

ABNE ☐☐☐☐
        7

GERNES ☐☐☐☐☐☐
      2

PATOOT ☐☐☐☐☐☐
      3

TAORRC ☐☐☐☐☐☐
        5

TEBE ☐☐☐☐
     10

LECYER ☐☐☐☐☐☐
       6

NOONI ☐☐☐☐☐
     9

☐☐☐☐☐☐   ☐☐☐☐☐☐
1 2 3 4 5 1 6   1 7 8 9 10 11

Fruit or Vegetable?

Circle all of the foods that are fruits.

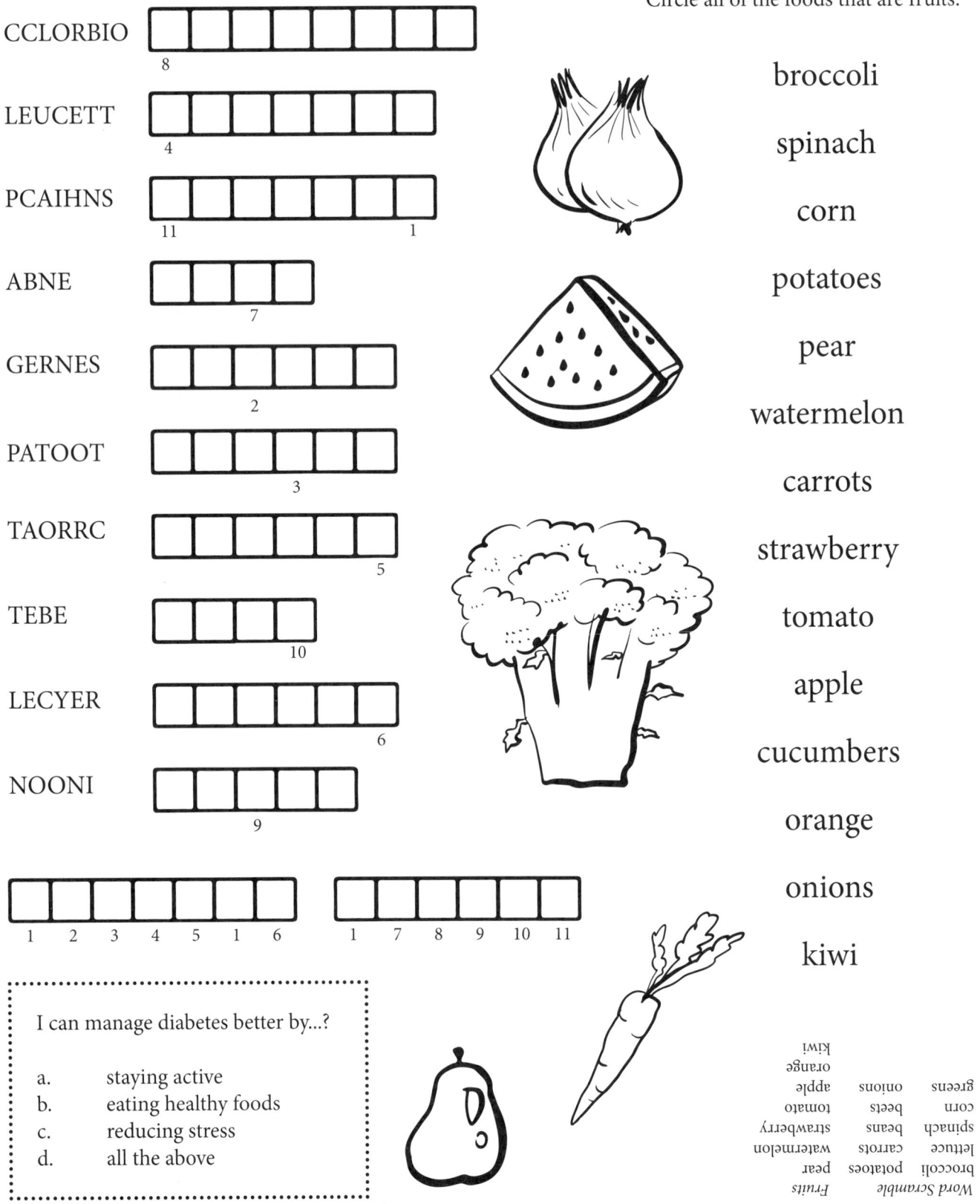

broccoli
spinach
corn
potatoes
pear
watermelon
carrots
strawberry
tomato
apple
cucumbers
orange
onions
kiwi

I can manage diabetes better by...?

a. staying active
b. eating healthy foods
c. reducing stress
d. all the above

Answer: d

Word Scramble
broccoli potatoes pear
lettuce carrots watermelon
spinach beans strawberry
corn beets tomato
greens onions apple
orange
kiwi

Fruits

Healthy Habits text by Floyd Stokes. Illustrations © Sheena Hisiro.

Match the fruit name to the picture.

CHERRY

APPLE

BANANA

ORANGE

GRAPES

LEMON

PINEAPPLE

STRAWBERRY

WATERMELON

Vegetables come from different parts of a plant. Write the part of the plant next to the vegetable.

Parts of Plants — Seed, Flower, Root, Leaf, Fruit, Stem, Bulb

Broccoli _____

Cauliflower _____

Tomato _____

Squash _____

Carrots _____

Onion _____

Celery _____

Asparagus _____

Lettuce _____

Spinach _____

Greens _____

Garlic _____

Okra _____

FUNNY CORNER

What did the one fruit say to the other fruit when their parents told them they could not get married?

We cantaloupe.

If you don't feel well, you should...?

a. fight through it
b. tell an adult
c. keep it to yourself
d. No Pain, no gain!

Answer: b

Seed — Okra, Cucumbers, Squash, Carrots
Flower — Broccoli, Cauliflower
Root — Carrots
Leaf — Lettuce, Spinach, Greens
Fruit — Tomato, Okra
Stem — Celery, Asparagus
Bulb — Onion, Garlic

Healthy Habits text by Floyd Stokes. Illustrations © Sheena Hisiro.

Fruit

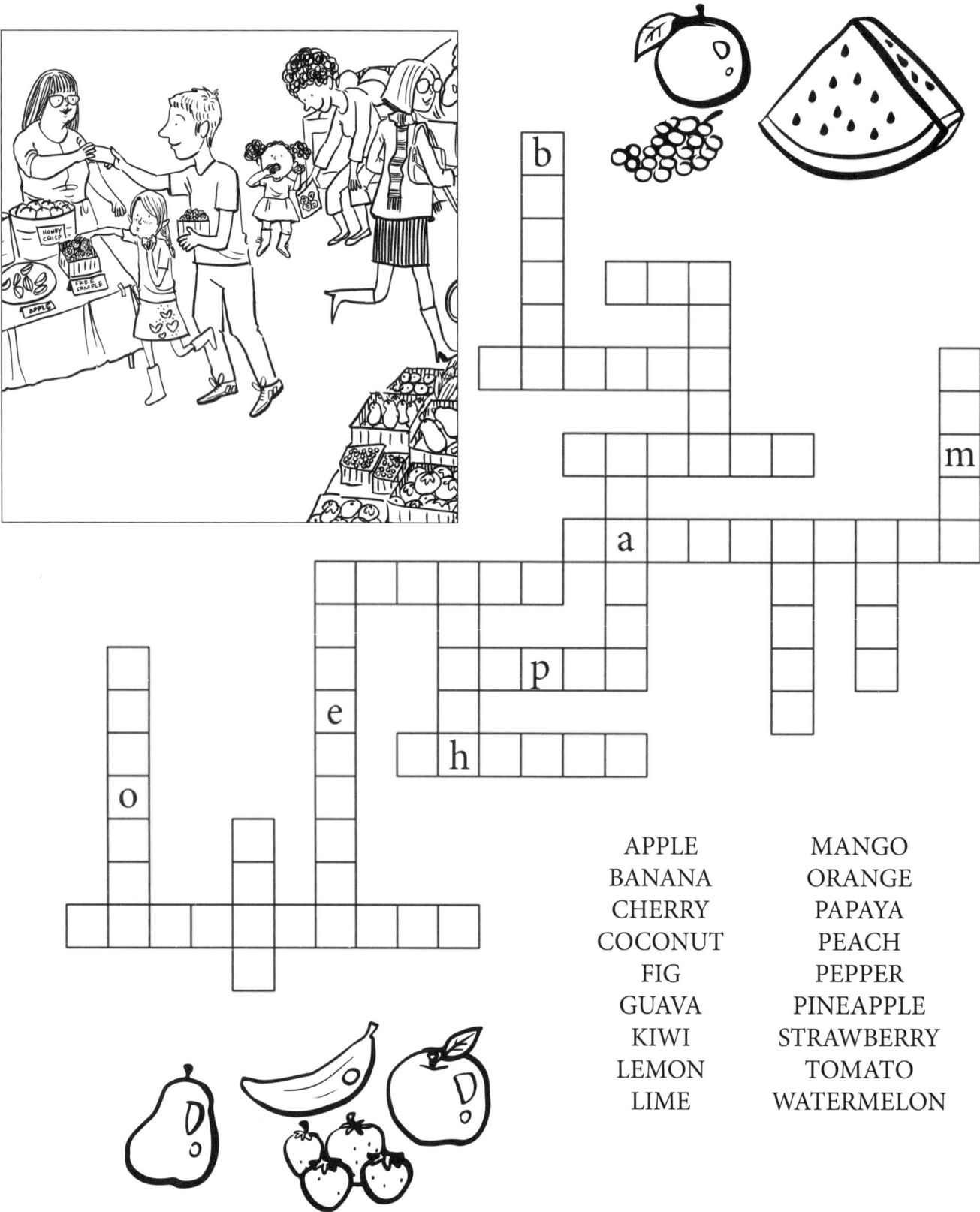

APPLE
BANANA
CHERRY
COCONUT
FIG
GUAVA
KIWI
LEMON
LIME
MANGO
ORANGE
PAPAYA
PEACH
PEPPER
PINEAPPLE
STRAWBERRY
TOMATO
WATERMELON

Answer: c

Help Tommy find his soccer ball.

START

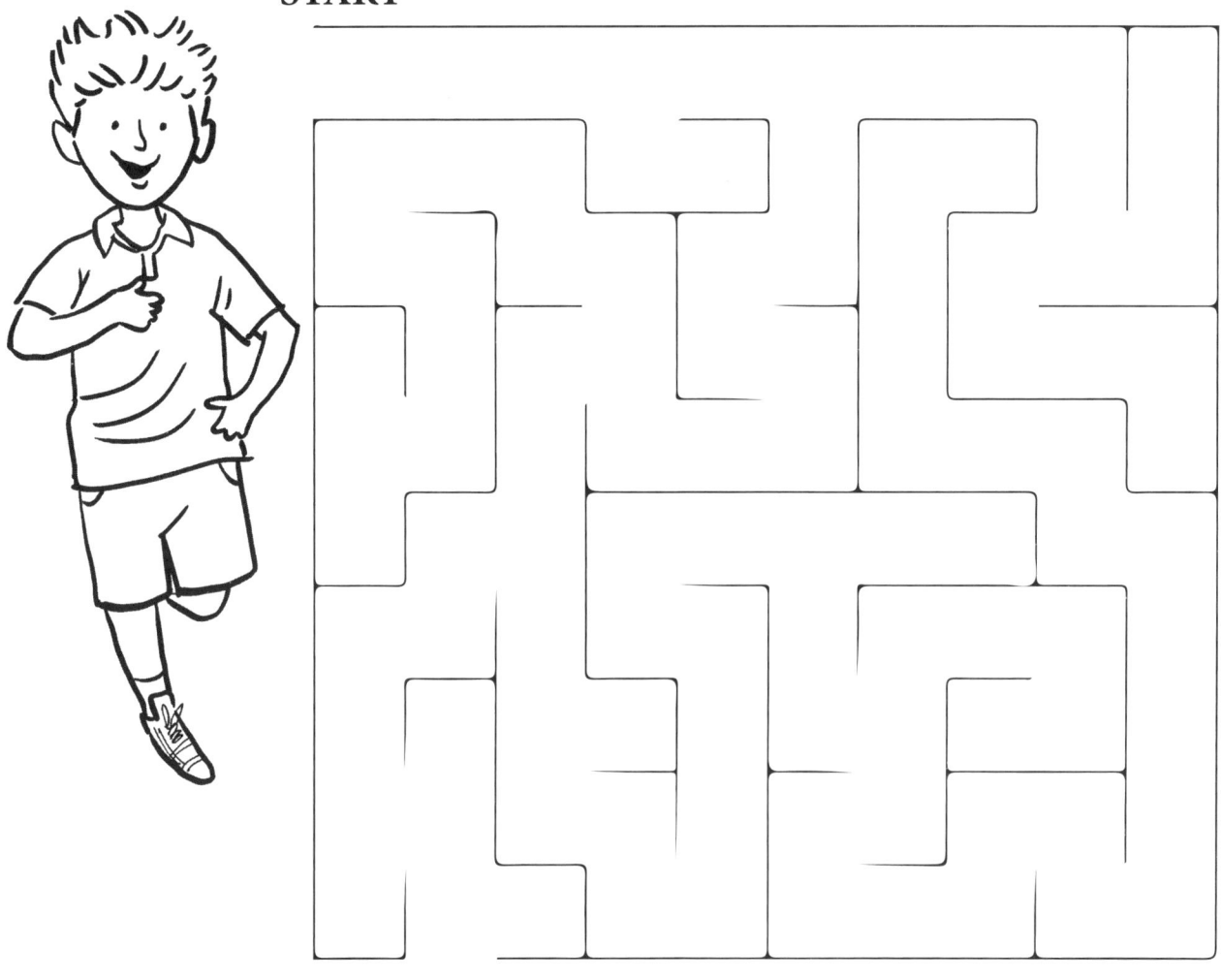

FINISH

What is the best way to fight diabetes?

a. play video games all day
b. watch TV all afternoon
c. play outside
d. stay in bed all day

FUNNY CORNER

What did the robber say at the bakery?

Give me all your dough.

What did the strawberry say to the raisin?

Help! I'm in a jam.

Answer: c

Healthy Habits text by Floyd Stokes. Illustrations © Sheena Hisiro.

Vegetables

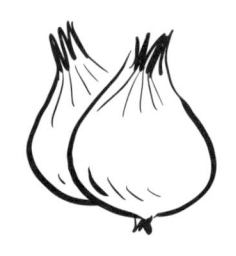

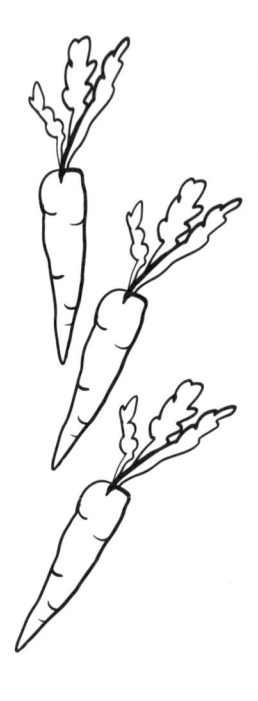

```
A B C E L E R Y S P I N A C H
O H I P P G G R E E N S T I B
E T G D U G E L S F W D R V Z
R K Q B M P B E E T S T M S T
M N I E P L B T Z D F P Y M R
F I N E K A R T I C H O K E S
P R P A I N O U S P R C W U S
F U J K N T C C C E E O G H G
M O K R A A C E M A L A D H R
O Q W O N I O N S F R T S W A
A D Z S A N L O I A K R A D R
A A V G N S I L P B L C O R N
S L V Y J G U S N I E X A T M
P L P E K A A E O C A E O S S
E T C U C U M B E R S O H I M
```

ARTICHOKES
BEETS
CAULIFOWER
CUCUMBERS
LETTUCE
PEAS
PUMPKIN
CARROTS
CORN
GREENS
ONIONS
PLANTAINS
ASPARAGUS
BROCCOLI
CELERY
EGGPLANT
OKRA
PEPPERS
SPINACH

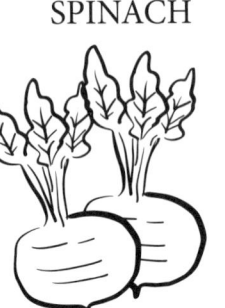

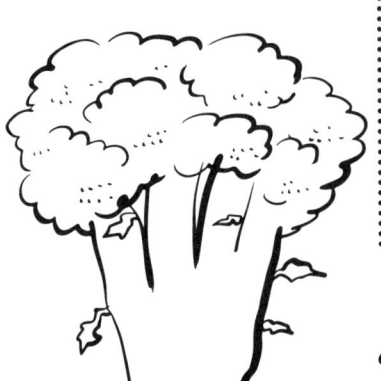

Glucose is a sugar that is the body's main source of...?

a. fuel
b. oxygen
c. water
d. red blood cells

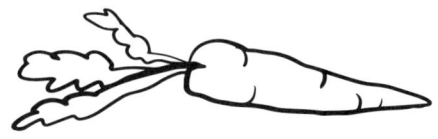

Answer: a

12 Healthy Habits text by Floyd Stokes. Illustrations © Sheena Hisiro.

Fun at the Park

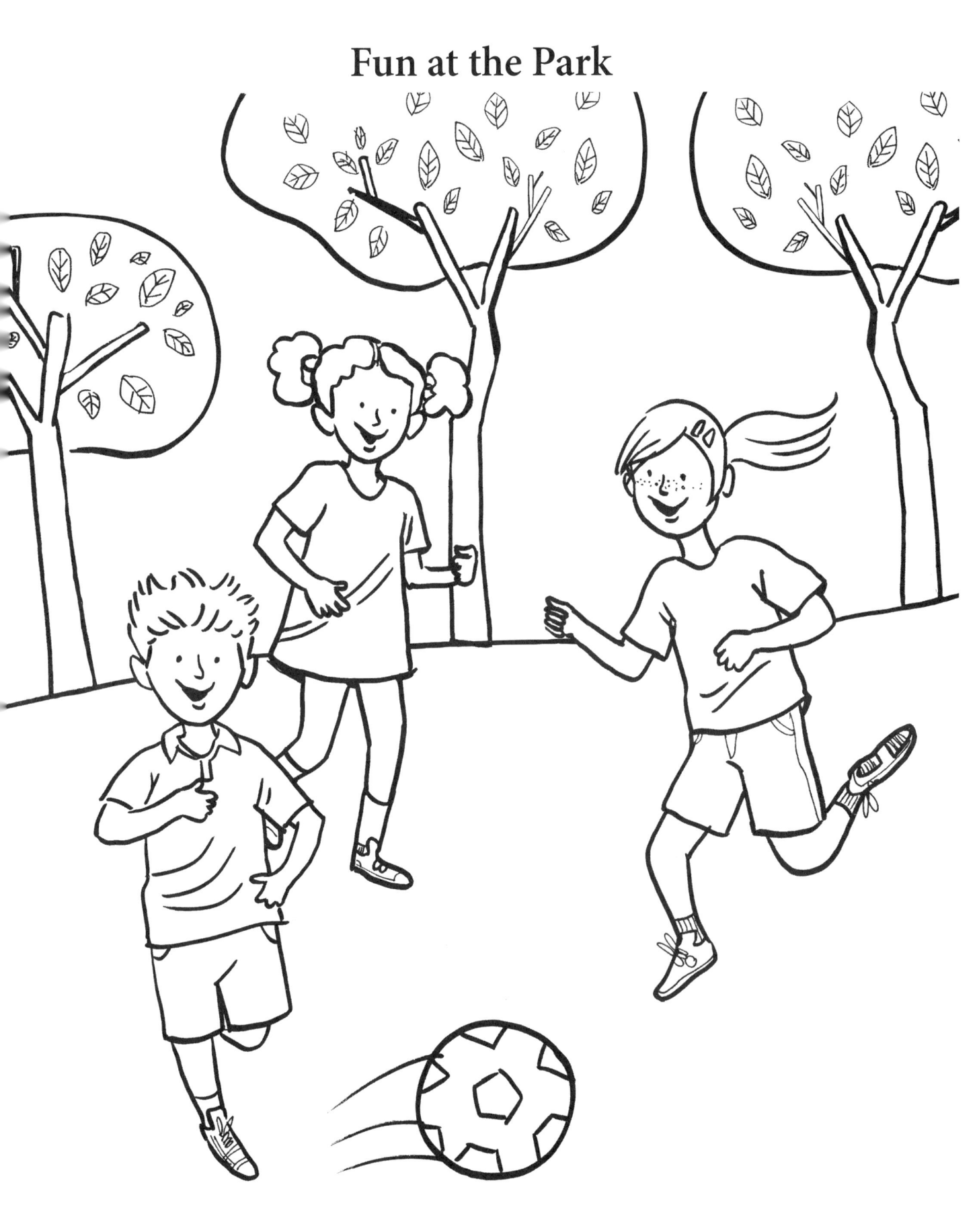

Healthy Habits text by Floyd Stokes. Illustrations © Sheena Hisiro.

Draw which comes next.

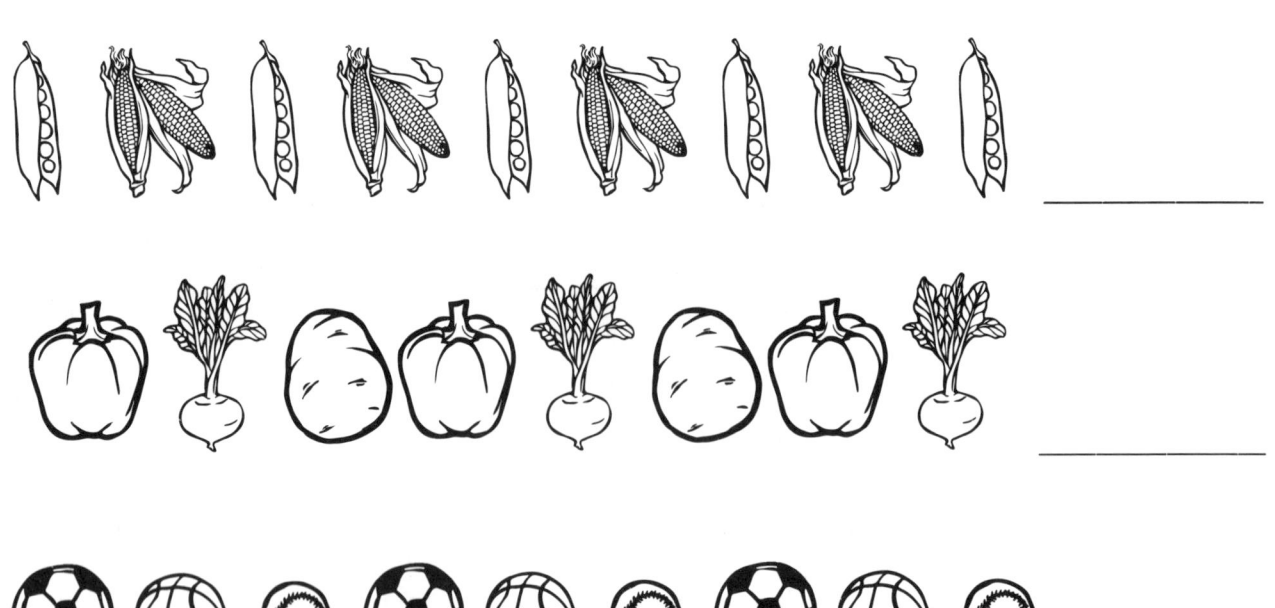

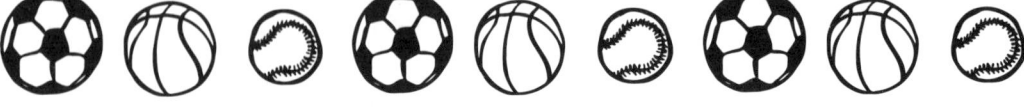

Crossword Puzzle

Use the words below to complete the crossword puzzle.

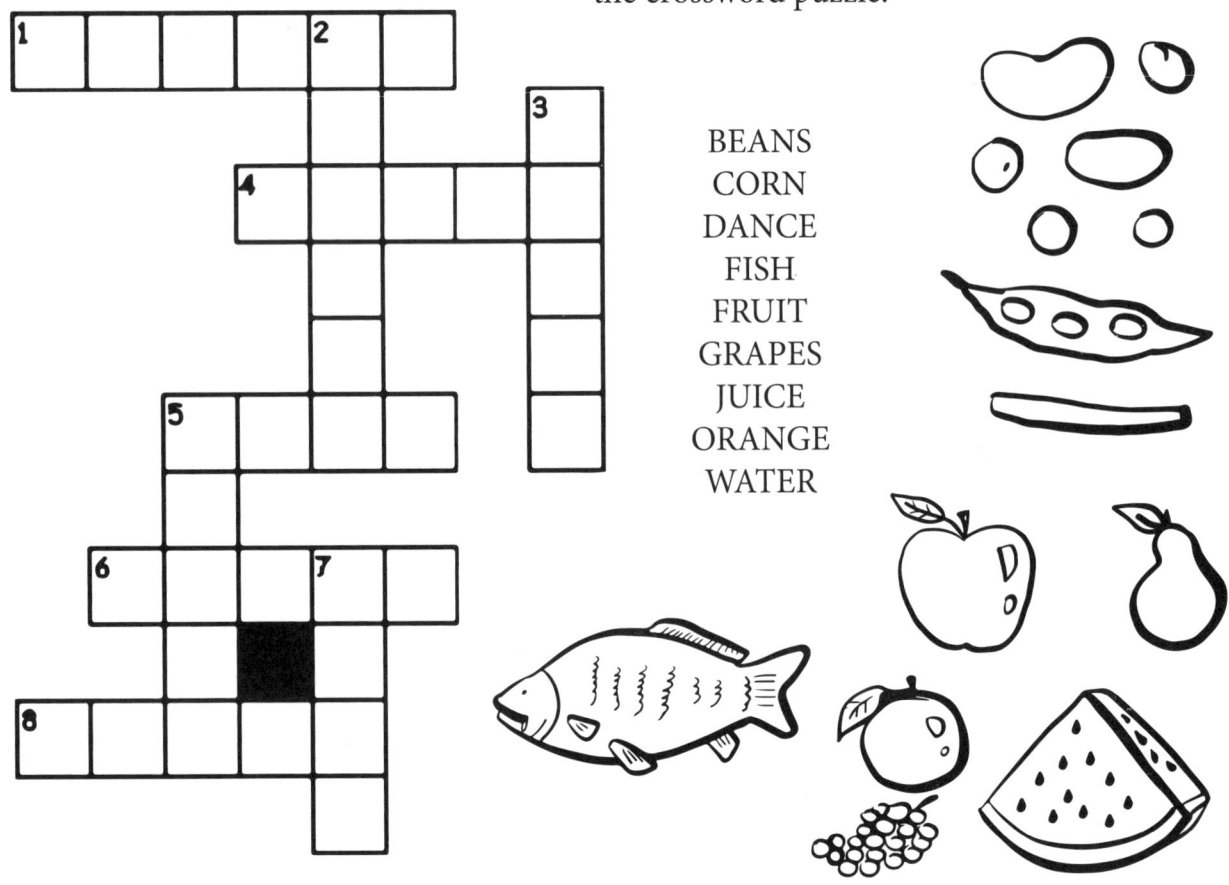

BEANS
CORN
DANCE
FISH
FRUIT
GRAPES
JUICE
ORANGE
WATER

14 *Healthy Habits text by Floyd Stokes. Illustrations © Sheena Hisiro.*

Fruit

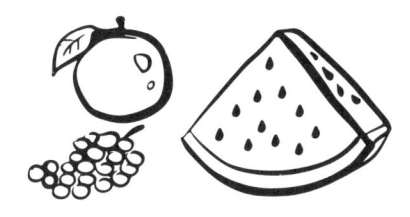

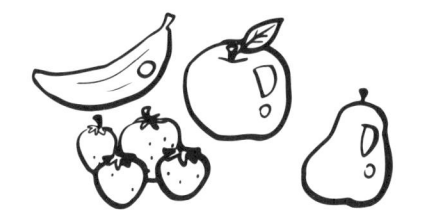

```
L E M O N A N I W I K X
X I E P A P A Y A E A N
G T M M A N G O B G S Y
I O P E A V A U G G T R
F M A P P L E E R T R R
W A T E R M E L O N A E
B T T U N O C O C M W H
B O R E P P E P V E B C
N Z H C A E P L F L E Y
Y H V E G N A R O O R H
P I N E A P P L E N R L
B A N A N A I Q Q R Y C
```

APPLE
CHERRY
GUAVA
LEMON
ORANGE
PEACH
STRAWBERRY
WATERMELON
BANANA
FIG
KIWI
MANGO
PAPAYA
PINEAPPLE
TOMATO

True or False

Only people with diabetes should watch what they eat.

FUNNY CORNER

What did the peach say to the doctor?

I can see but things are kind of fuzzy.

What did the fruit say to the other fruit when he heard they were going to the fair?

Kiwi go too?

Answer: False because all people should make healthy choices.

Healthy Habits text by Floyd Stokes. Illustrations © Sheena Hisiro.

Complete the dot-to-dot activities.

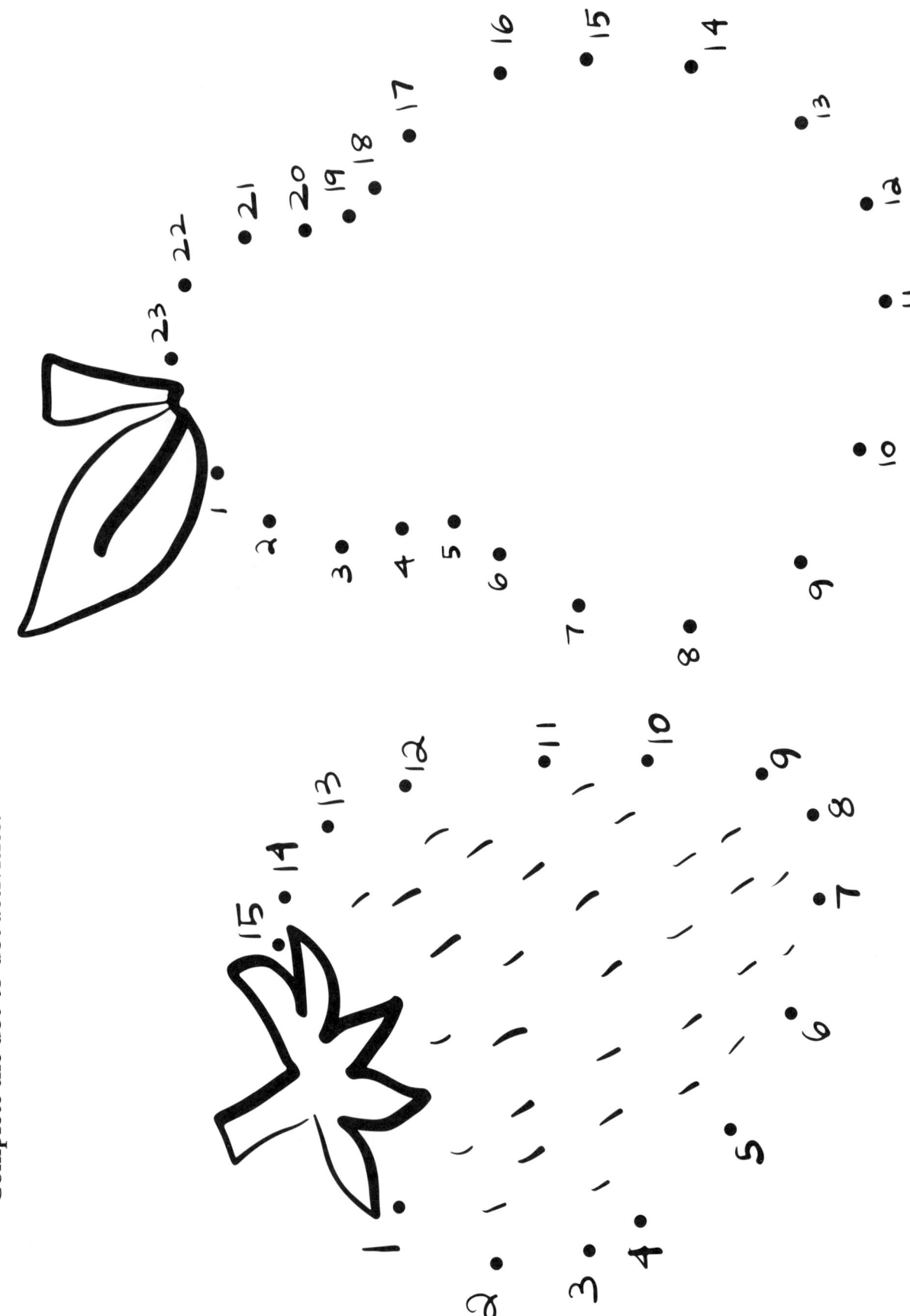

FRUIT SQUARES

EXAMPLE:

Taking turns, connect a line from one apple to another. Whoever makes the line that completes a box writes his initials inside the box. Each box is worth 1 point. Boxes with a star are worth 5 bonus points. Boxes with watermelon are worth 10 bonus points. The person with the most points at the end wins!

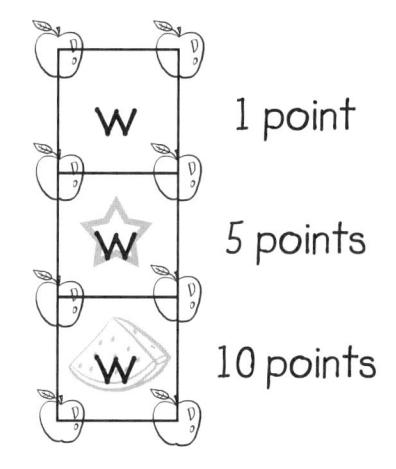

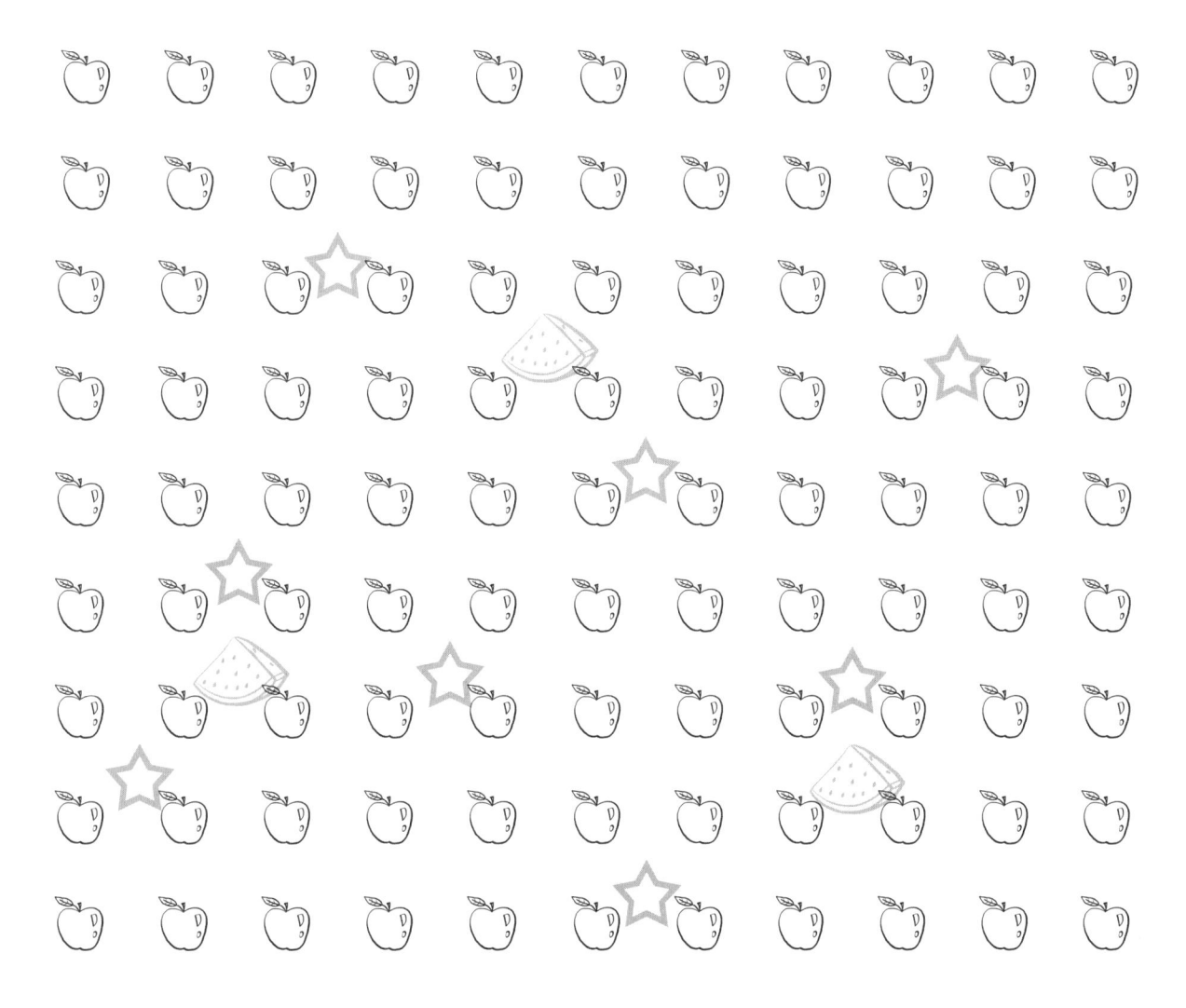

Red, White, and Blue Smoothies

Submitted by Capital BlueCross

Ingredients (serves 2)
2 cups plain greek yogurt
1/2 cup low-fat milk
1 1/2 cups (8 oz) blueberries
1/4 teaspoon vanilla extract
raspberries (garnish)

Directions
Blend yogurt, milk, and vanilla. Pour half the vanilla smoothie into two glasses. Add blueberries to the remaining smoothie mixture and blend. Pour over the vanilla smoothie in the glasses. Top with fresh raspberries.

Nutritional Facts (per serving)
Calories: 303 Total Fat: 9.6g Sat. Fat: 5.9g Protein: 11.5g

Berries are great sources of antioxidants, which help fight disease. Blueberries are one of the most powerful antioxidants. A variety of berries is available at local farmers markets throughout the summer months. This smoothie contains more than 100% of the daily recommended allowance of vitamin C.

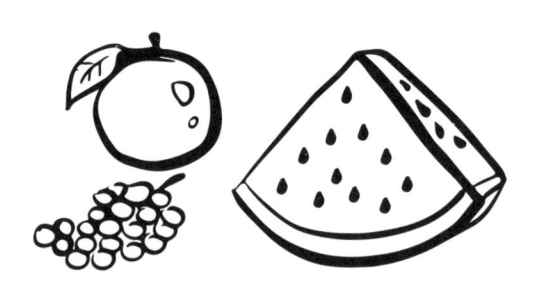

FUNNY CORNER

Which fruit is always signing autographs?

Star fruit

How much fruit should children eat during snack time?

a. about a 1/4 cup
b. about a 1/2 cup
c. about 1 cup
d. about 2 cups

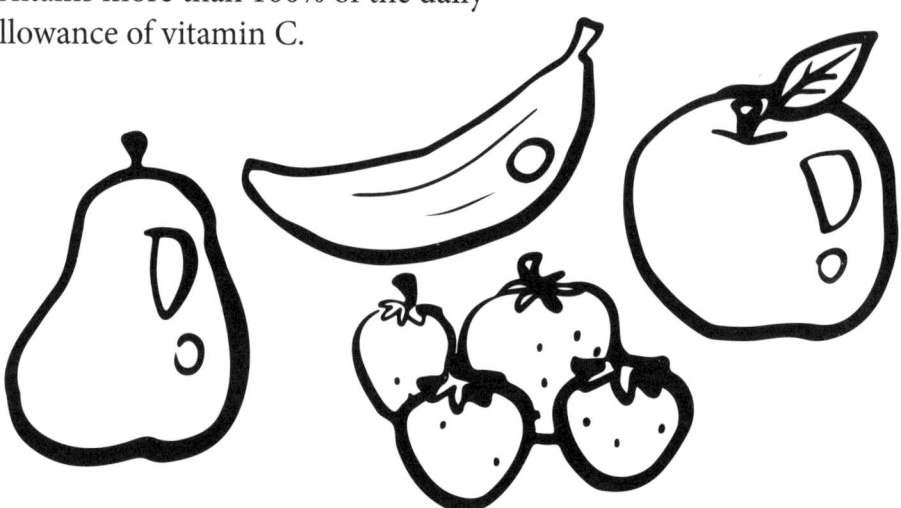

Answer: b

Healthy Habits text by Floyd Stokes. Illustrations © Sheena Hisiro.

Complete the dot-to-dot activity. Then, draw your favorite fruits for a smoothie inside.

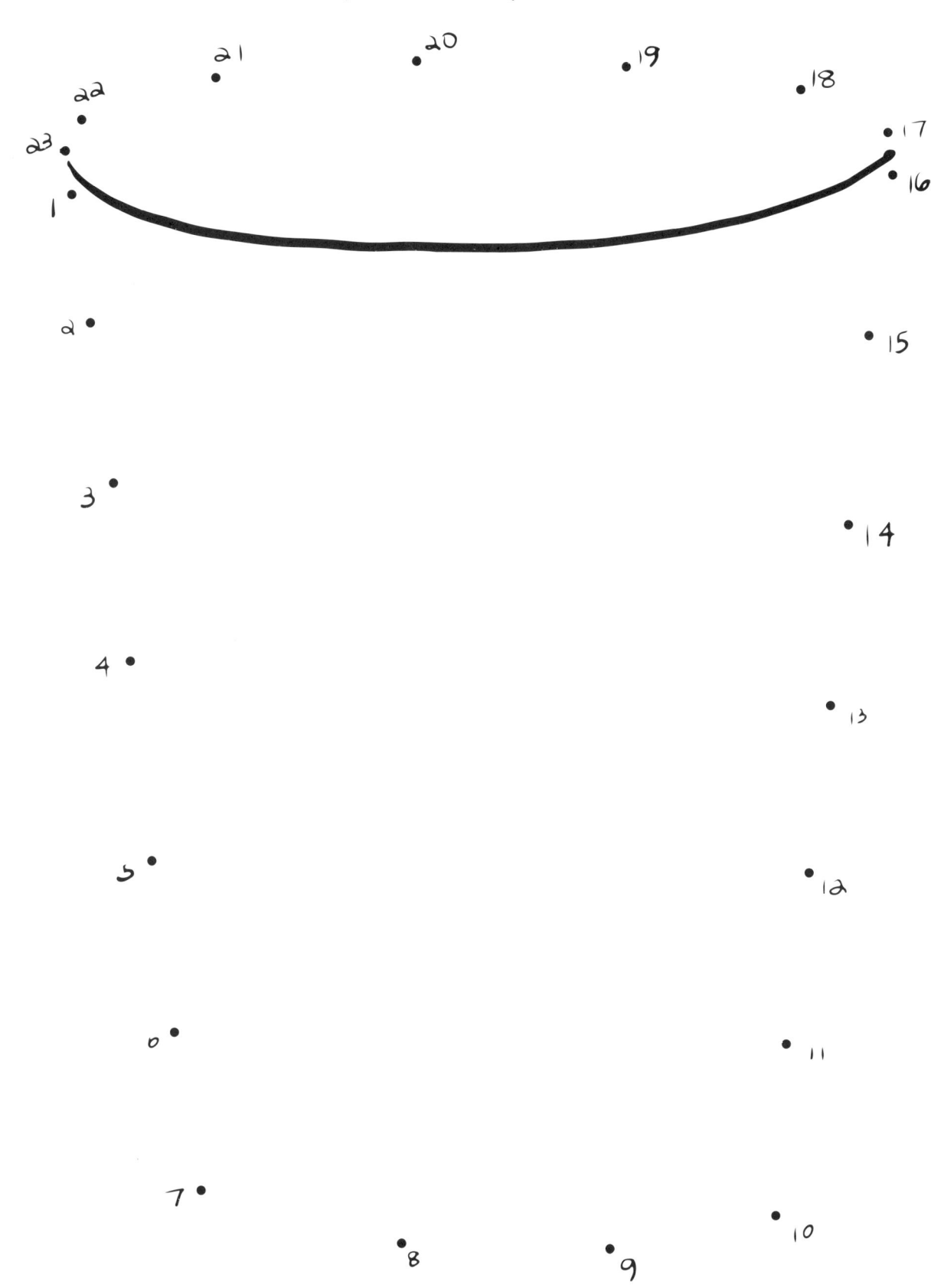

Healthy Habits text by Floyd Stokes. Illustrations © Sheena Hisiro.

Dairy

Say Cheese!

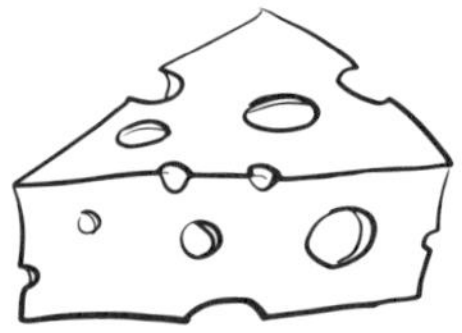

```
C O L B Y F A M E R I C A N
L R T L E E E I L T M L X O
A T M I S T S N M G O U D A
T C R S Q A C P O Z Z M G F
W B I E H Z E R N C Z U Z T
A W C S F P U O T P A E J C
S I O Q Q A G V E A R N N S
O S T M H R R O R E E S A N
T O T U O M U L E O L T F C
N X A G O E Y O Y E L E U C
P T G H B S E N J E A R J O
C H E D D A R E A U J P P J
I E Z T I N E K C M S V R G
F Z S S S L X V K I W I C C
```

AMERICAN   BRIE   CHEDDAR
COLBY   COTTAGE   FETA
GORGONZOLA GOUDA   GRUYERE
MONTEREY JACK MOZZARELLA MUENSTER
PARMESAN   PROVOLONE   RICOTTA

Diabetes is a disease in which there is usually too much...?

a. salt in the blood
b. sugar in the blood
c. sugar in the heart
d. salt in the heart

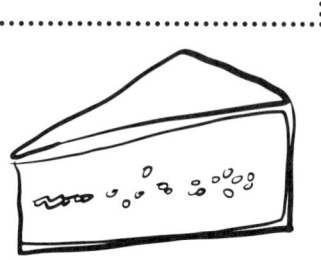

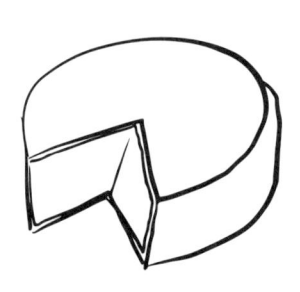

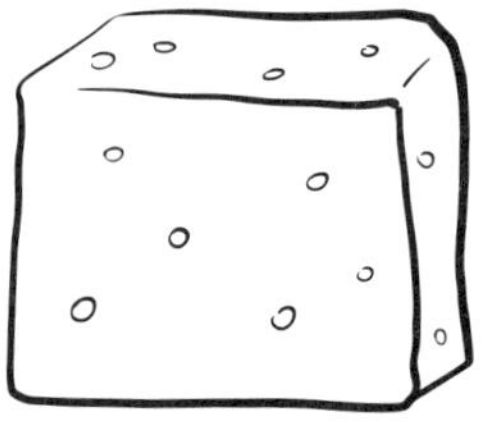

Answer: b

Healthy Habits text by Floyd Stokes. Illustrations © Sheena Hisiro.

Dairy, Healthy Oils and Fats

Oils are not a food group, but they do provide essential nutrients. However, only small amounts of oils are recommended. That's because they still contain calories. Therefore, the amount of oils and solid fats needs to be limited.

There is another special category called empty calories. They include foods with solid fats and/or added sugars. They provide no nutritional value and should only be eaten on occasion.

> The pancreas is a long, flat gland in your belly that helps your...?
>
> a. lungs breath
> b. legs run fast
> c. helps your body digest food
> d. eyes see better

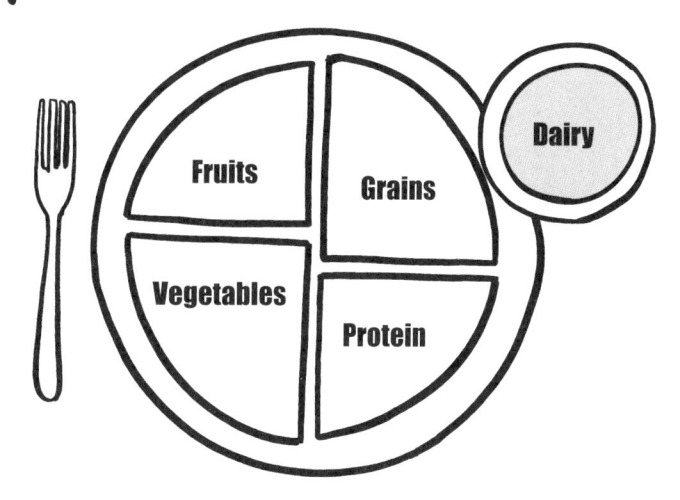

Match each word or picture with the correct food group.

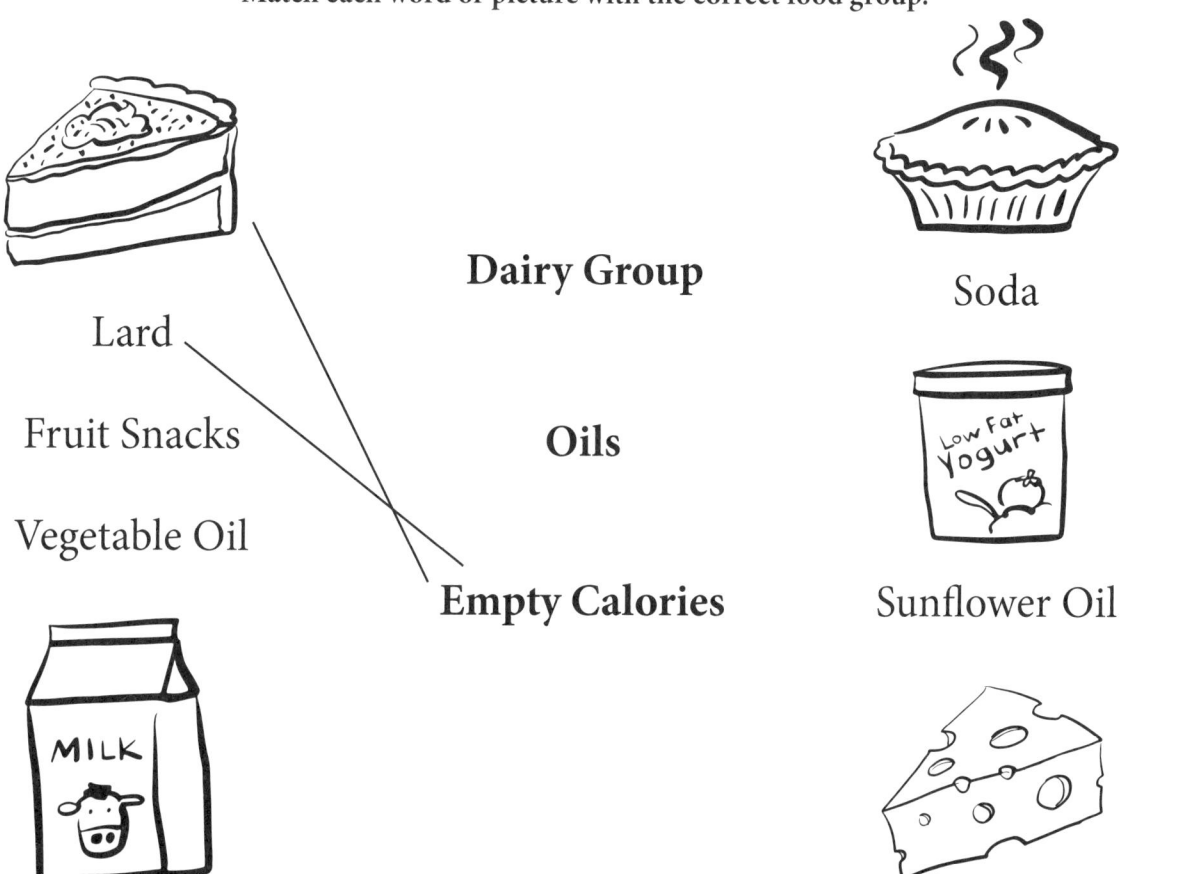

Dairy Group

Lard

Fruit Snacks

Oils

Vegetable Oil

Empty Calories

Soda

Sunflower Oil

Healthy Habits text by Floyd Stokes. Illustrations © Sheena Hisiro.

Answer: c

Circle the item in each row that doesn't belong.

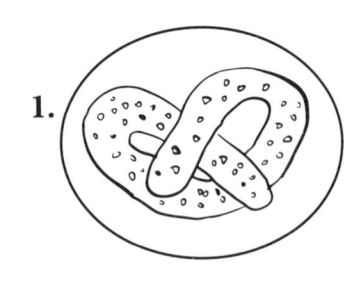

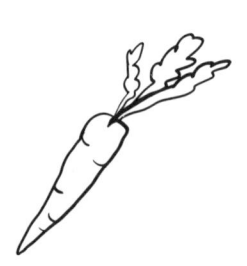

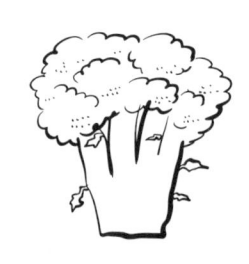

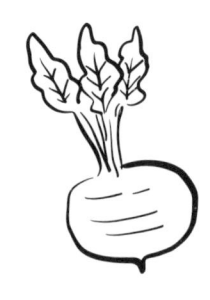

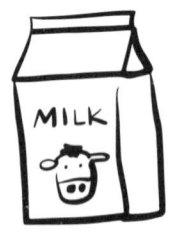

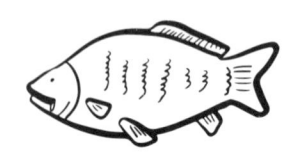

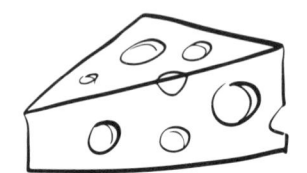

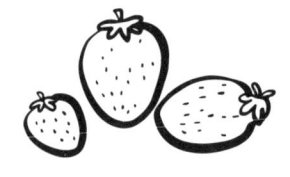

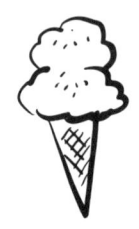

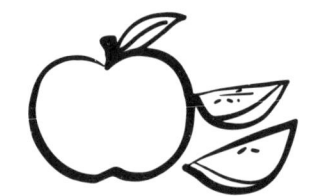

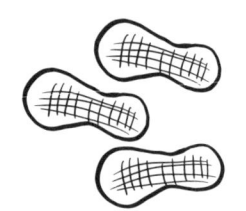

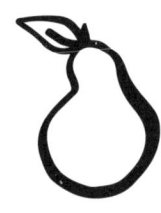

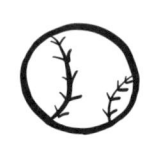

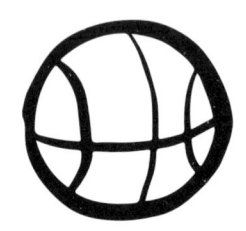

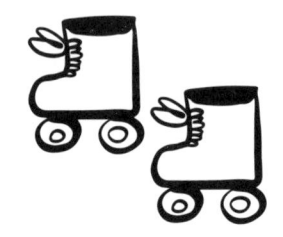

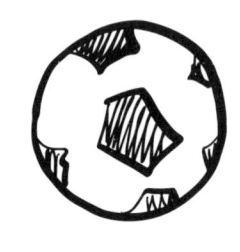

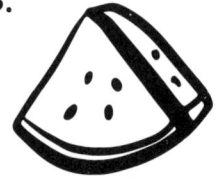

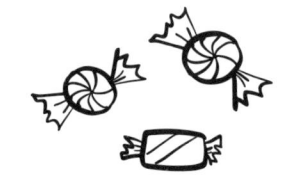

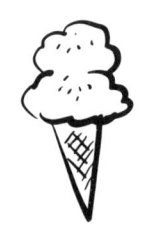

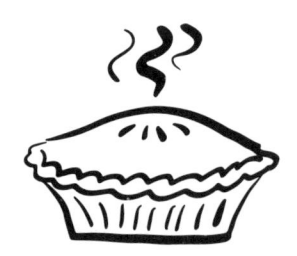

1.
2.
3.
4.
5.

Proteins

All foods made from meat, poultry, seafood, beans and peas, eggs, processed soy products, nuts, and seeds are considered protein. Beans and peas have protein but are also part of the Vegetable Group.

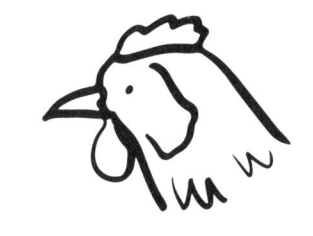

Where do they come from?
Match the food with the animal it comes from.

Beef	Sheep
Ham	Deer
Lamb	Pig
Pork	Calf
Veal	Chicken
Venison	Pig
Poultry	Cow

FUNNY CORNER

What did the one fruit say to the other fruit?

We make a good pear.

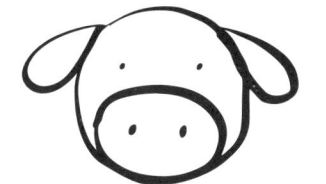

Which is the most common form of diabetes?

a. Type 1
b. Type 2
c. Type 3
d. Type 4

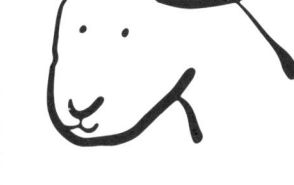

Which are not a kind of bean or pea that you can eat?

Black Beans
Garbanzo Beans
Kidney Beans
Blue Beans
Lima Beans
Navy Beans
Pinto Beans
Soy Beans
Army Beans
Black-Eyed Peas

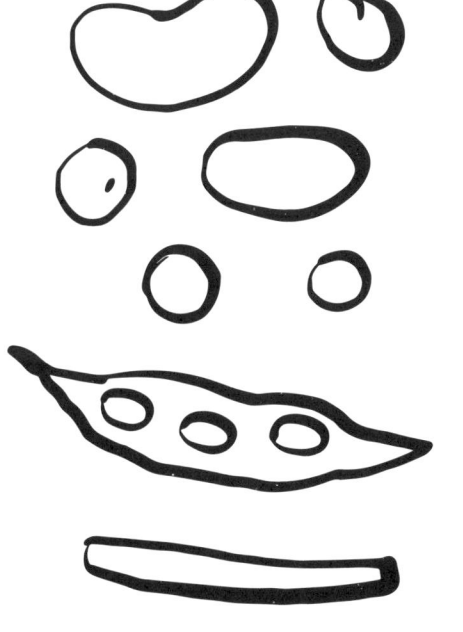

Orange Beans
Chickpeas
Split Peas
White Beans
Lentils
Mexican Jumping Beans
Fava Beans
Cranberry Beans
Pink Beans

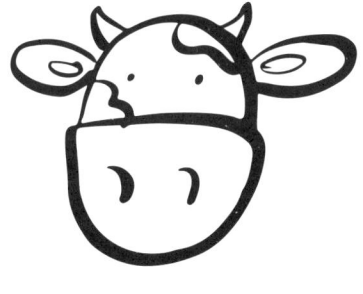

Not Beans or Peas
Mexican Jumping Beans
Blue Beans
Orange Beans
Army Beans

Where do they come from?
Beef - Cow
Ham - Pig
Lamb - Sheep
Pork - Pig
Veal - Calf
Venison – Deer
Poultry - Chicken

Answer: b

Healthy Habits text by Floyd Stokes. Illustrations © Sheena Hisiro.

Facts about Fats

There are good fats and bad fats. Your body needs good fats to:

1. give your body energy
2. support cell growth
3. protect your organs
4. keep your body warm
5. help your body absorb some nutrients
6. and produce important hormones

Bad fats are typically solid at room temperature. Good fats are typically liquid at room temperature. Circle the good fats.

Sunflower Oil	Chicken Fat
Milk Fat	Canola Oil
Cottonseed Oil	Shortening
Lard	Soybean Oil
Safflower Oil	Beef Fat
Butter	Olive Oil
Corn Oil	Margarine

What color are they?

Carrot	Black
Cucumber	White
Lemon	Purple
Plum	Brown
Tomato	Green
Berries	Orange
Cauliflower	Red
Pinto Beans	Blue
Olives	Yellow

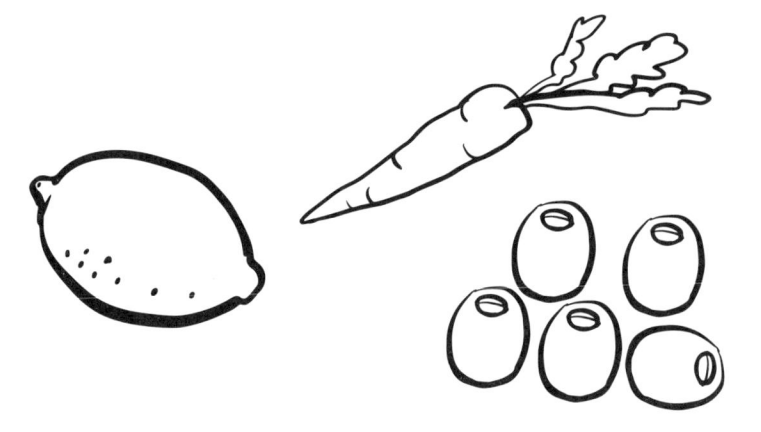

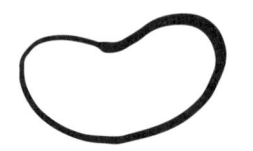

FUNNY CORNER

While performing at the circus, the apple tumbled, orange peeled and the banana spit.

What did the salad children say to the salad parents?

Please lettuce go with you.

Diabetes is a disease that affects how the body uses...?

a. air
b. glucose
c. salt
d. fat

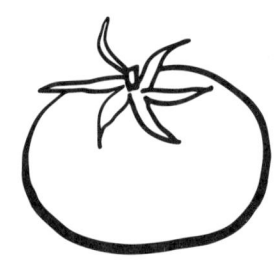

What Color?
Carrots – orange
Lemon – yellow
Brown – pinto beans
Tomatoes – red
White - cauliflower
Blue – berries
Purple – grapes
Black – olives
Green - cucumber

Good oils
Canola Oil
Corn Oil
Cottonseed Oil
Olive Oil
Safflower Oil
Soybean Oil
Sunflower Oil

Answer: b

Healthy Habits text by Floyd Stokes. Illustrations © Sheena Hisiro.

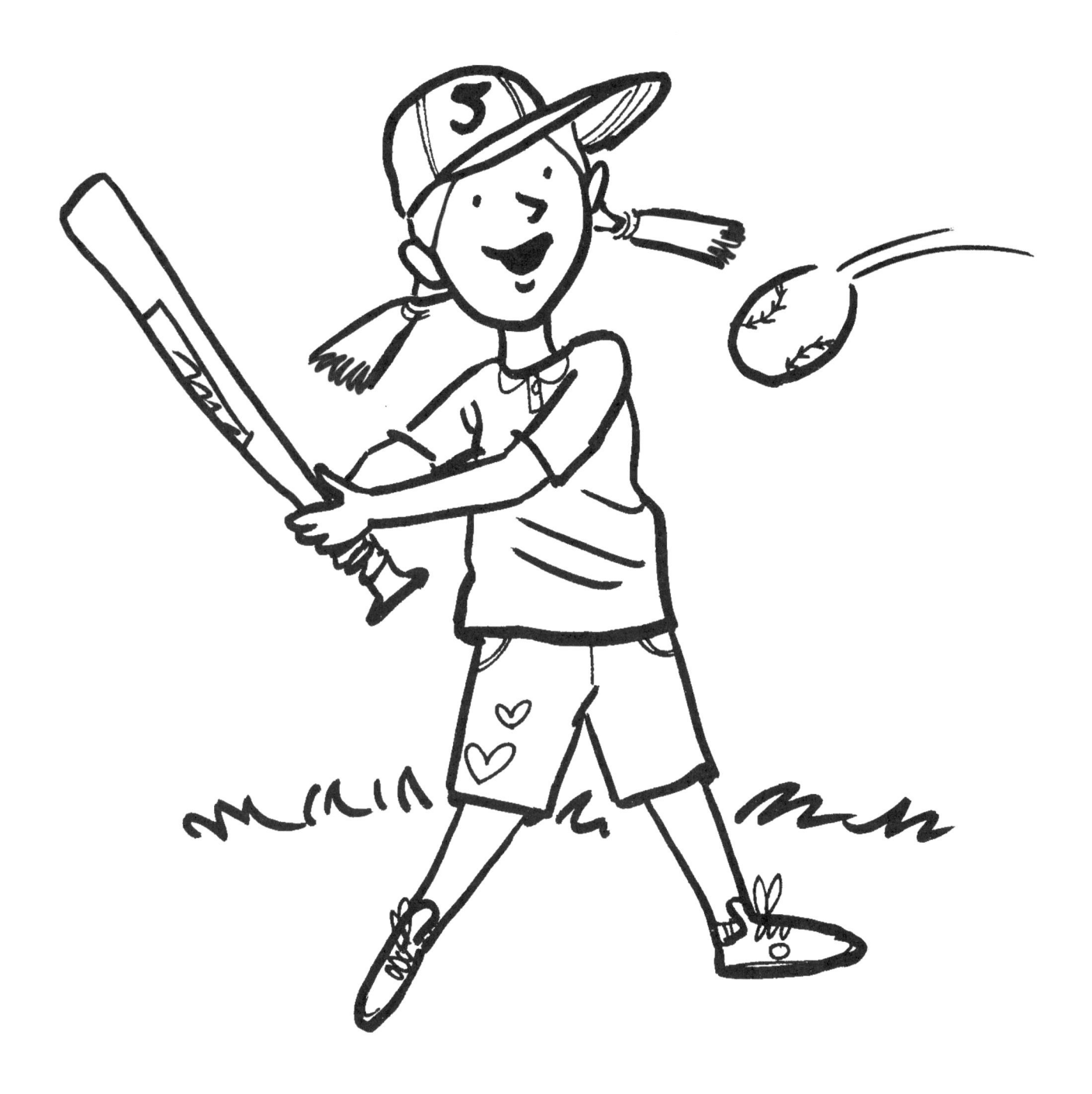

Staying active is important for...?

a. everyone
b. just kids with diabetes
c. just kids who love sports
d. just boys

FUNNY CORNER

Which cheese is good at playing basketball?

Colby

Answer: a

Healthy Habits text by Floyd Stokes. Illustrations © Sheena Hisiro.

Seafood

Seafood is a nutrient rich food that is a good source of protein, vitamins and minerals. Scientific studies continue to explore the relationship between the unique type of fat found in seafood, the omega-3 fatty acids DHA and EPA, in the prevention or mitigation of common chronic diseases.

Below is a list of seafood. Some are finfish and some are shellfish. Circle the shellfish.

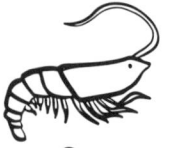

Octopus
Haddock
Shrimp
Trout
Mussels
Salmon

Catfish
Oysters
Tuna
Crayfish
Snapper
Flounder

Crab
Squid
Clams
Lobster
Scallops

FUNNY CORNER

Which fish has good rhythm?

A Snapper

Which fish likes to fight all the time?

Sword fish

_____ provide no real nutritional value other than calories, they should be limited.

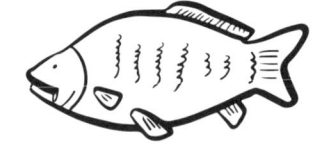

a. vegetables
b. sweets
c. fruits
d. chicken

A Secret Morse Code
Use the key below to solve the puzzle.

A •-   B -•••   C -•-•   D -••   E •   F ••-•   G --•   H ••••   I ••   J •---   K -•-   L •-••   M --

N -•   O ---   P •--•   Q --•-   R •-•   S •••   T -   U ••-   V •••-   W •--   X -••-   Y -•--   Z --••

___ ___ ___ ___ ___ ___ ___ ___ ___ ___ ___
•-   ••••   •   •-••   -   ••••   -•--   -••   ••   •   -   ••   •••

___ ___ ___
-   ••••   •

___ ___ ___ ___ ___ ___ ___ ___
-•   ••••   •   •••   •-   --   •   ••-•   ---   •-•

___ ___ ___ ___ ___ ___ ___ ___ ___
•   ••••-   •   •-•   -•--   ---   -•   •

Answer: b

Shellfish
octopus
oysters
clams
scallops
crab
squid
crayfish
lobster
shrimp
mussels

Morse Code
A healthy diet is the same for everyone.

Healthy Habits text by Floyd Stokes. Illustrations © Sheena Hisiro.

Staying Active

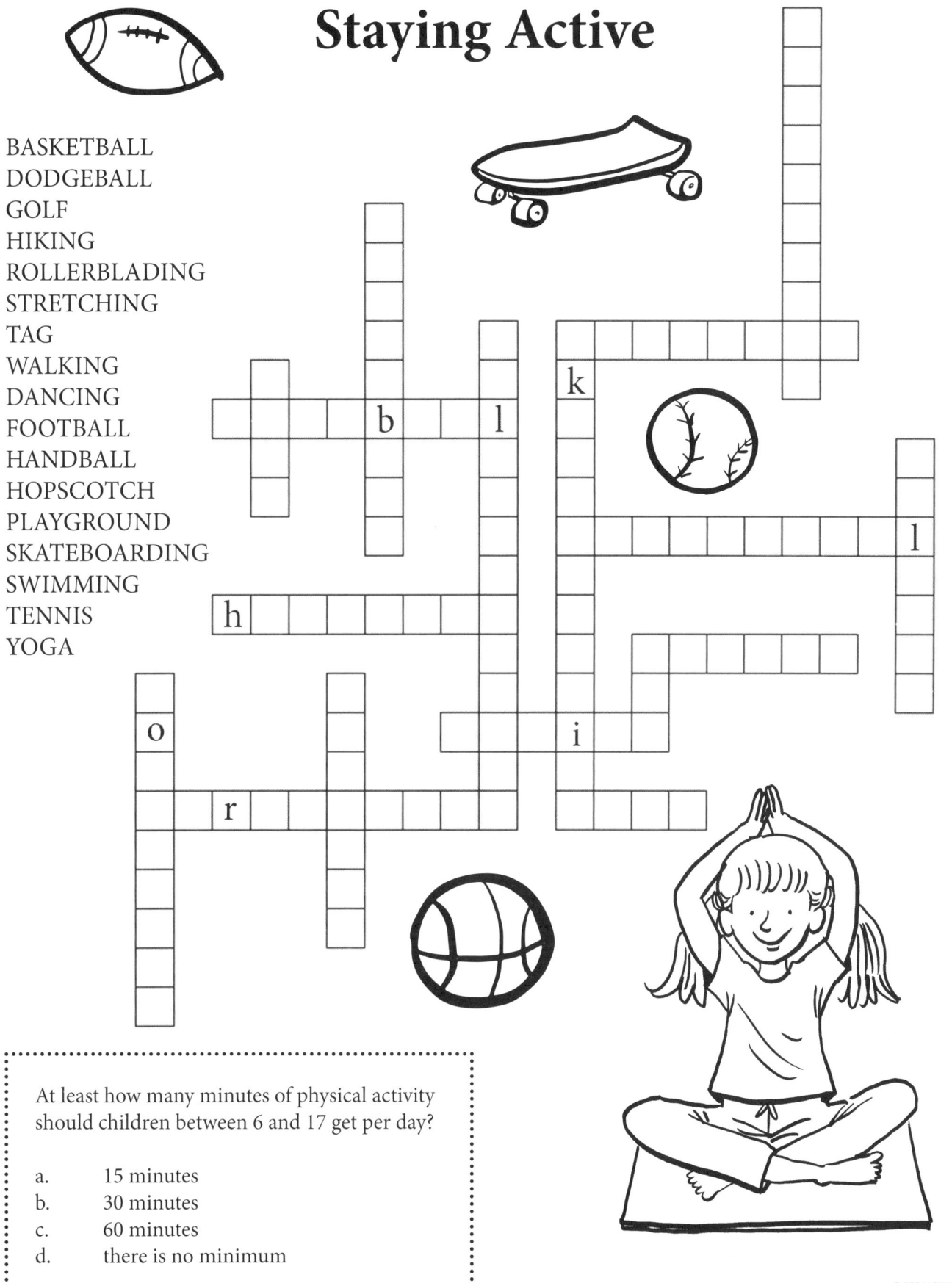

BASKETBALL
DODGEBALL
GOLF
HIKING
ROLLERBLADING
STRETCHING
TAG
WALKING
DANCING
FOOTBALL
HANDBALL
HOPSCOTCH
PLAYGROUND
SKATEBOARDING
SWIMMING
TENNIS
YOGA

At least how many minutes of physical activity should children between 6 and 17 get per day?

a. 15 minutes
b. 30 minutes
c. 60 minutes
d. there is no minimum

Answer: c

Healthy Habits text by Floyd Stokes. Illustrations © Sheena Hisiro.

Grains and Protein Foods Group

MyPlate has five food groups that make up a healthy diet. Proteins and grains are needed for a balanced diet.

When ordering food at a restaurant, avoid...?

a. jumbo
b. giant
c. super size
d. all the above

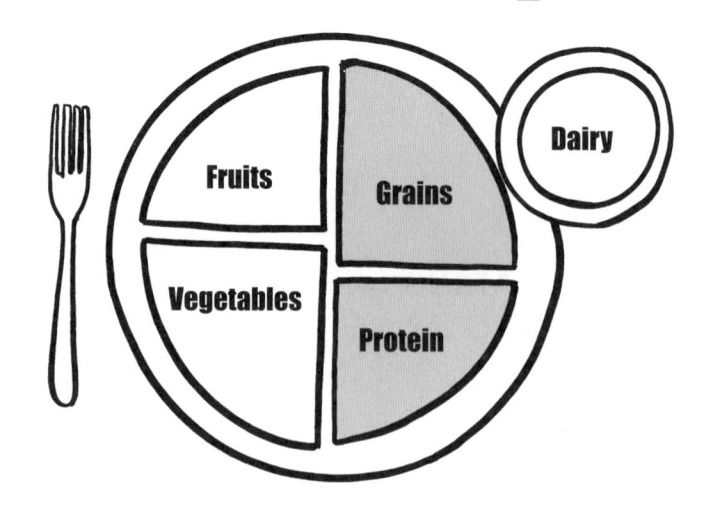

Match each word or picture with the correct food group.

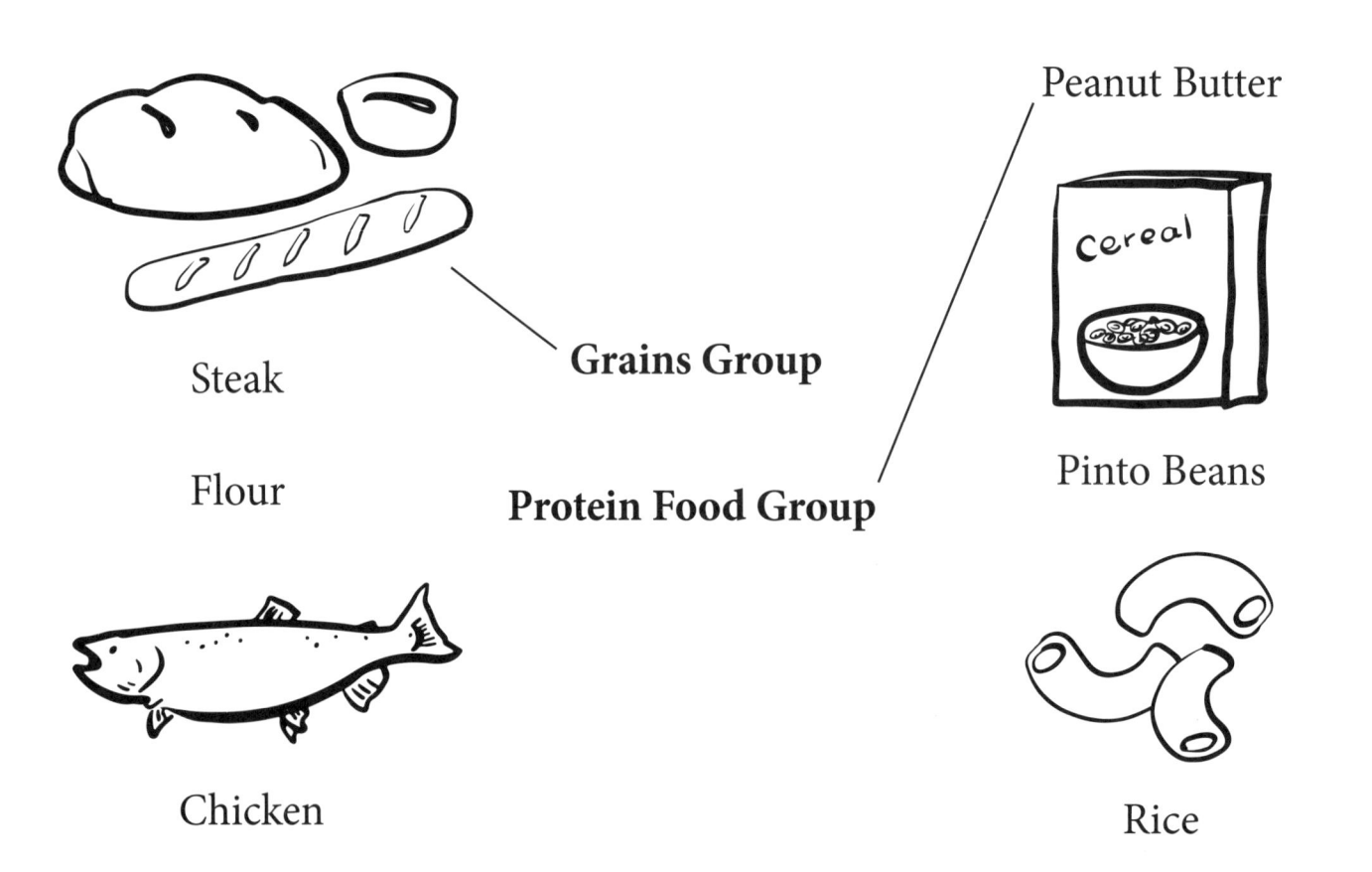

Steak

Flour

Chicken

Grains Group

Protein Food Group

Peanut Butter

Pinto Beans

Rice

Answer: d

Healthy Habits text by Floyd Stokes. Illustrations © Sheena Hisiro.

Grains

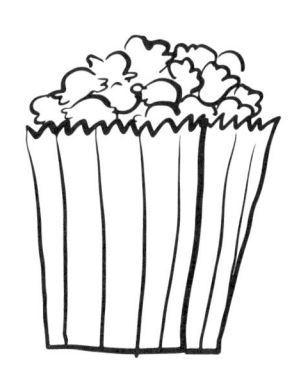

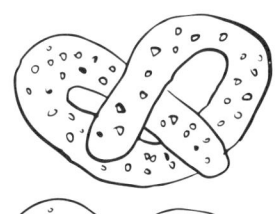

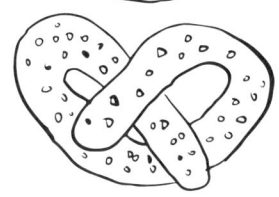

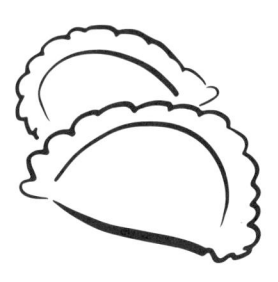

```
E I O O X E E A N L D E E I
E S E T B U C K W H E A T R
E D P O P C O R N E N F O S
Z G W R S N R I P S O T R R
B R E A D O N A L O O S T C
A A T I P O M A C U D E I P
O I B A R L E Y D K L O L A
P N S A E M A C E R E A L S
R I C E T E L E R J S R A T
J A G A Z C O U S C O U S A
M Z O E E M S T B X A M D T
C F Y H L N R J H X T M E A
G R I T S N Z K R J S I P N
C S A L G C I M V E S M G N
```

BARLEY
CEREALS
CRACKERS
MACARONI
OATS
POPCORN
RYE

BREAD
CORNMEAL
GRAIN
NOODLES
PASTA
PRETZELS
TORTILLAS

BUCKWHEAT
COUSCOUS
GRITS
OATMEAL
PITAS
RICE

When a person first has diabetes, he may…?

a. pee a lot
b. drink and eat a lot
c. feel tired
d. all the above

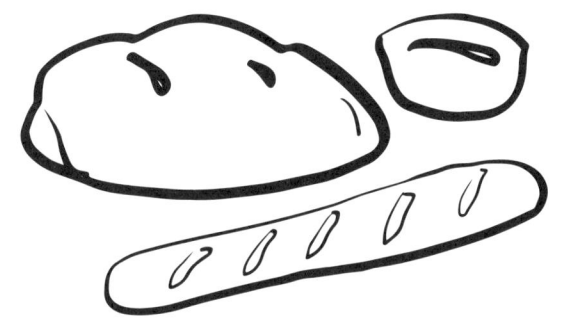

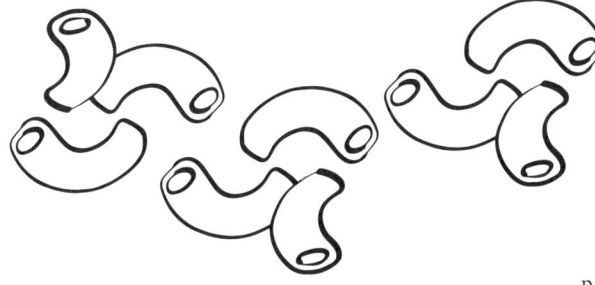

Answer: d

Healthy Habits text by Floyd Stokes. Illustrations © Sheena Hisiro.

Spot the Difference

There are 10 differences between these two pictures. Can you spot them?

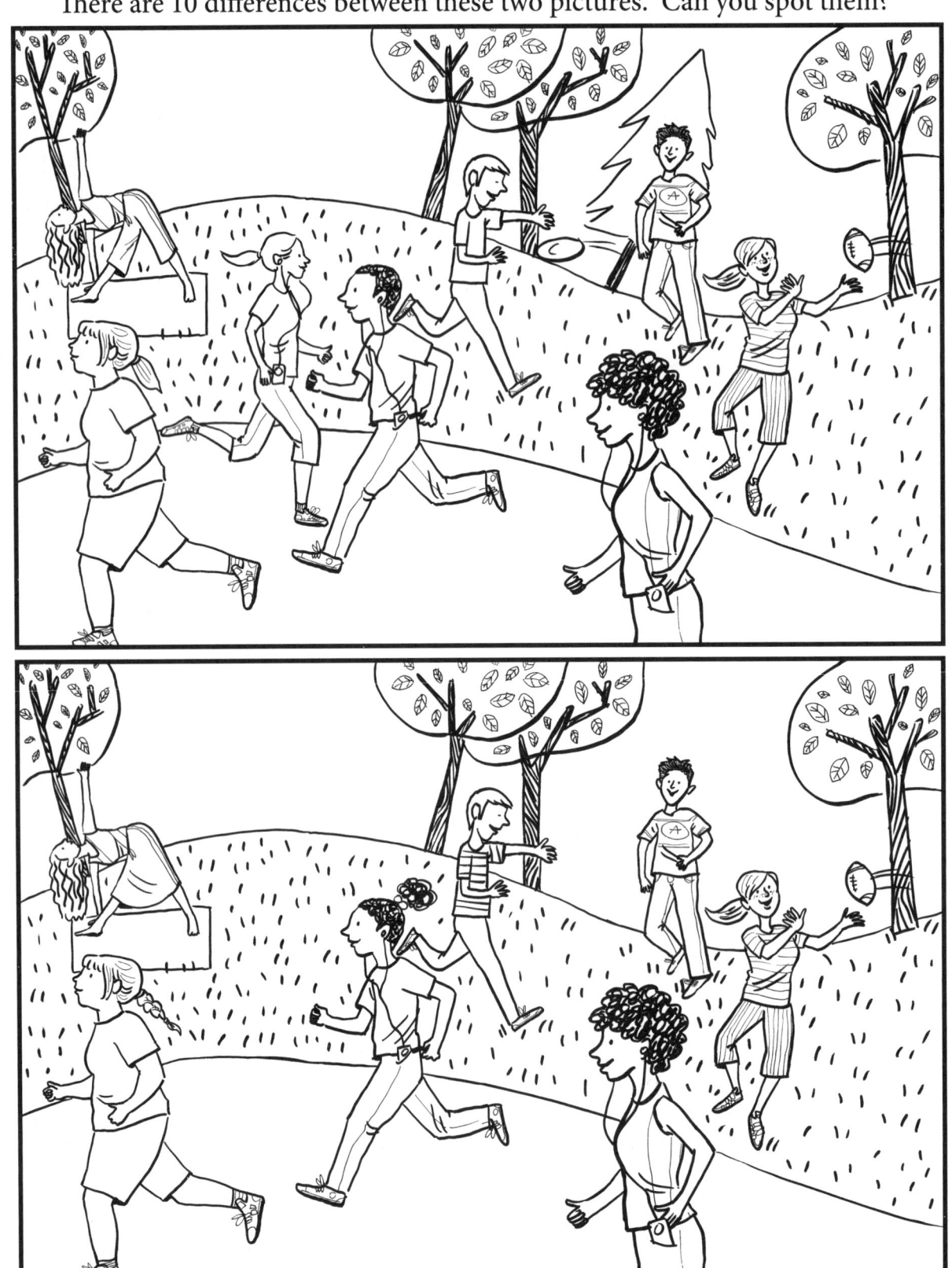

Healthy Habits text by Floyd Stokes. Illustrations © Sheena Hisiro.

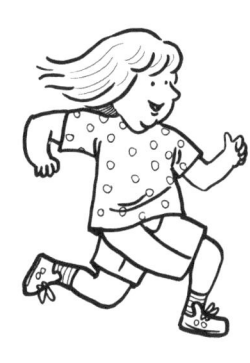

It's dinner time! Help Katy find her way to a balanced meal.

START

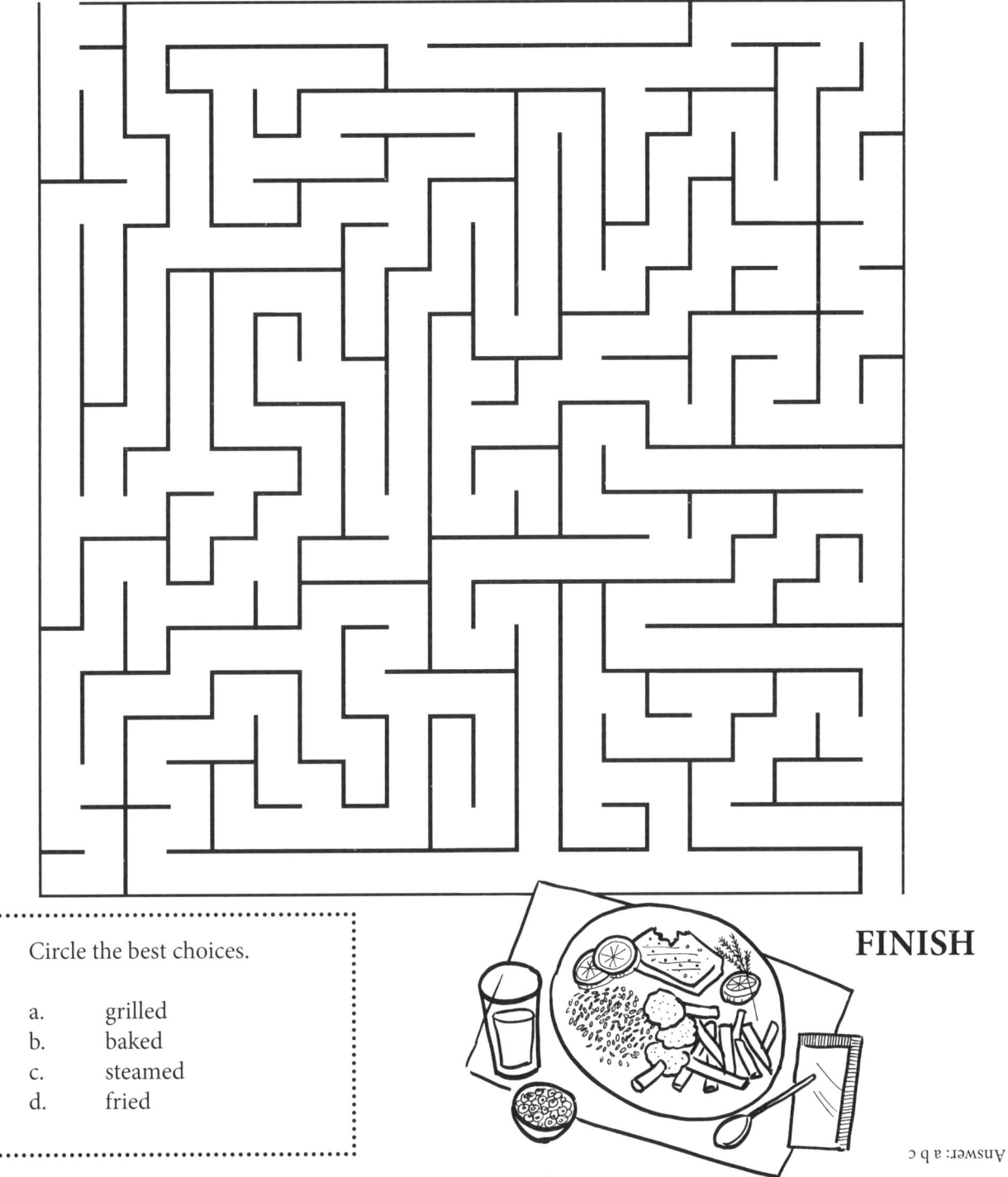

FINISH

Circle the best choices.

a. grilled
b. baked
c. steamed
d. fried

Answer: a b c

Healthy Habits text by Floyd Stokes. Illustrations © Sheena Hisiro.

Fun at the Farmer's Market

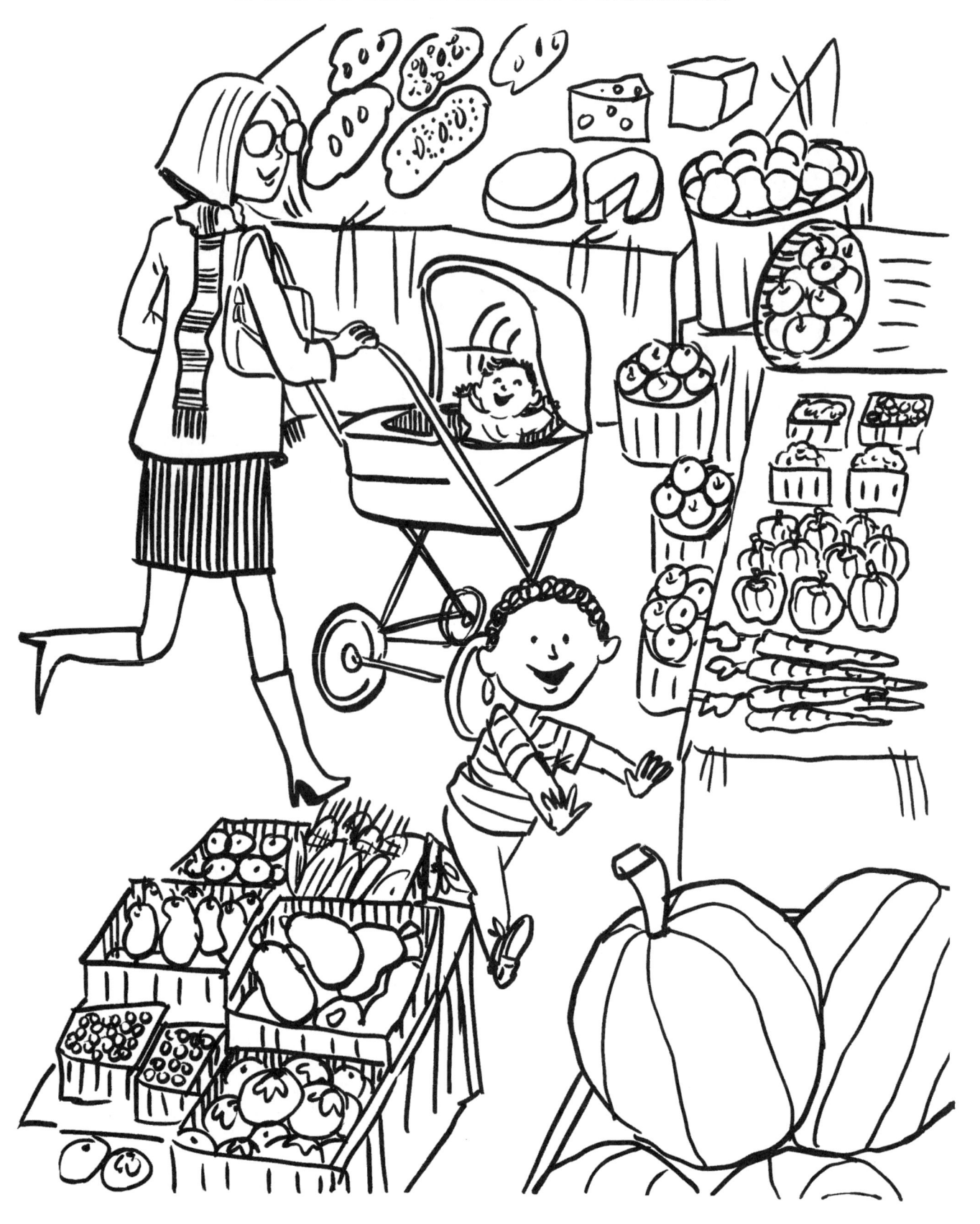

Healthy Habits text by Floyd Stokes. Illustrations © Sheena Hisiro.

Follow the trail to find out what activity each kid is doing.
Write the number below each object.

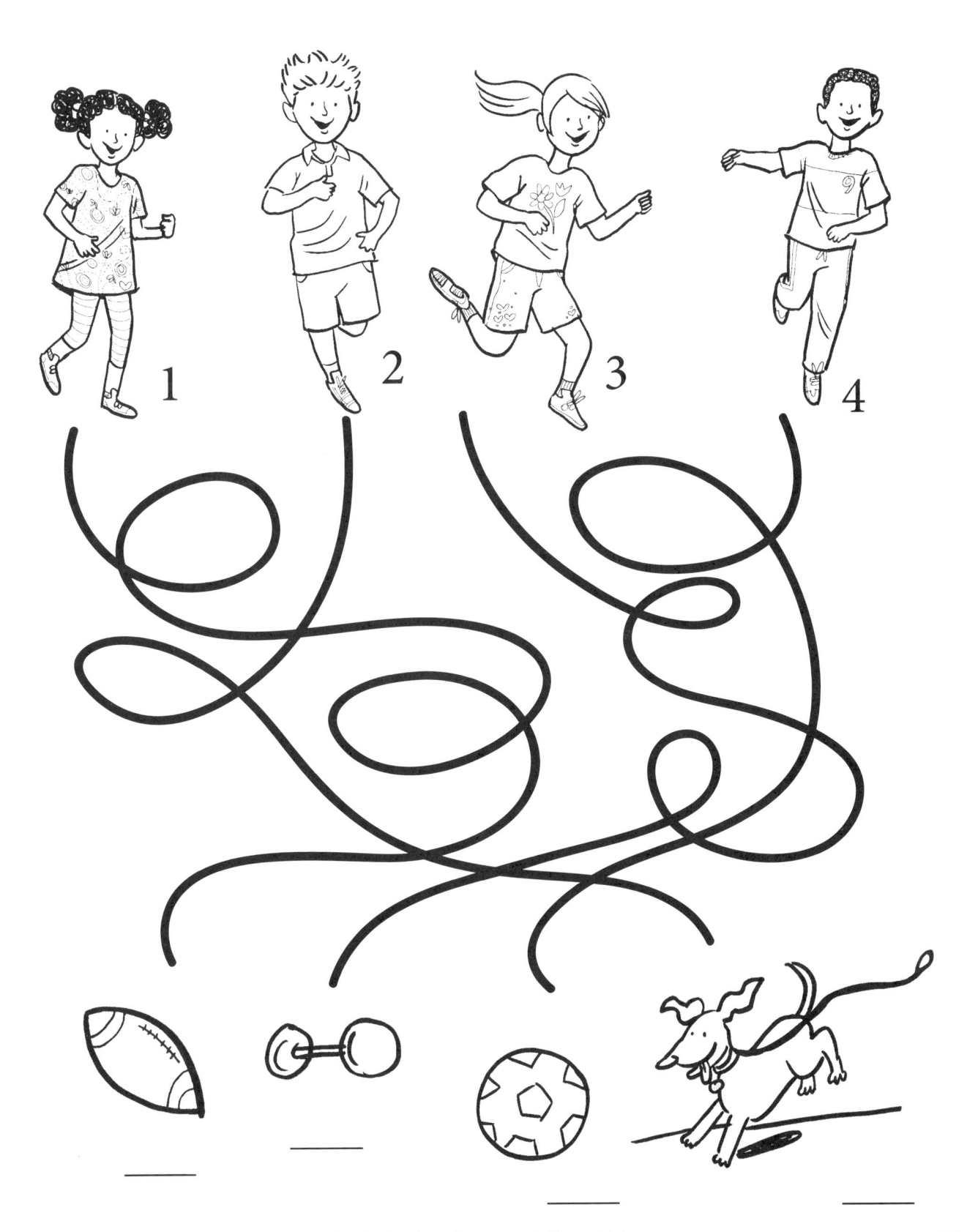

Healthy Habits text by Floyd Stokes. Illustrations © Sheena Hisiro.

Draw which comes next.

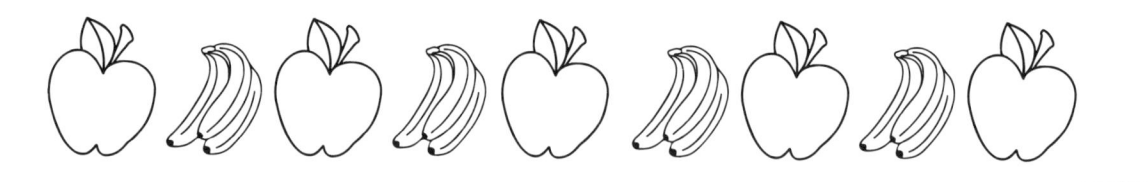

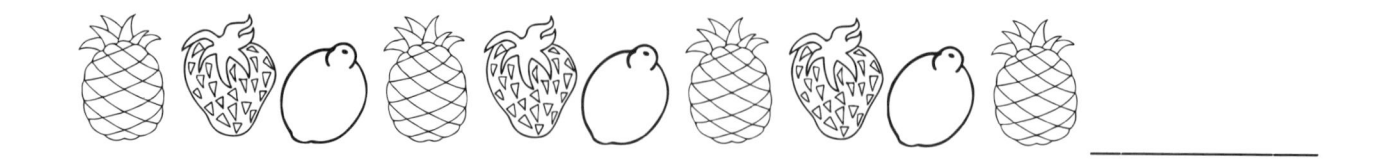

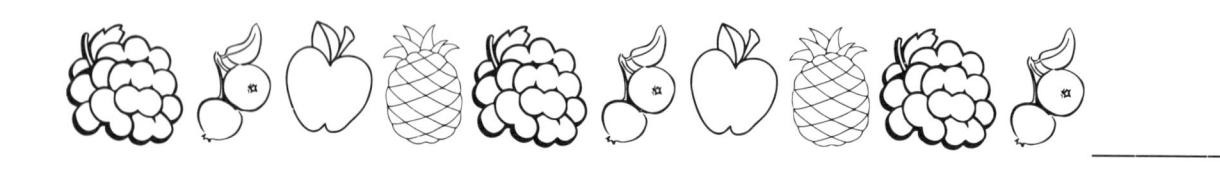

Word Search

Find the words in the puzzle below.

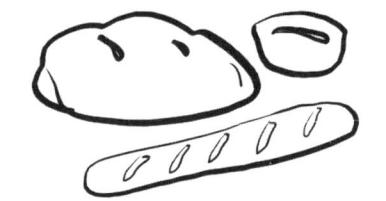

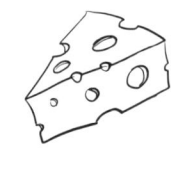

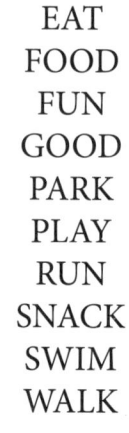

```
C R K O S D S J
T E A T F U N Y
Q B P A R K A X
F O O D U O C K
H F Z K N U K G
W A L K Y D R O
L D C S W I M O
V B P L A Y R D
```

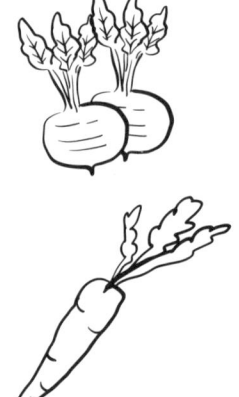

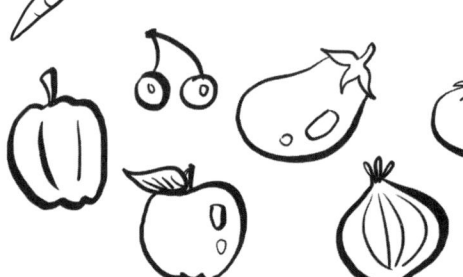

EAT
FOOD
FUN
GOOD
PARK
PLAY
RUN
SNACK
SWIM
WALK

Crossword

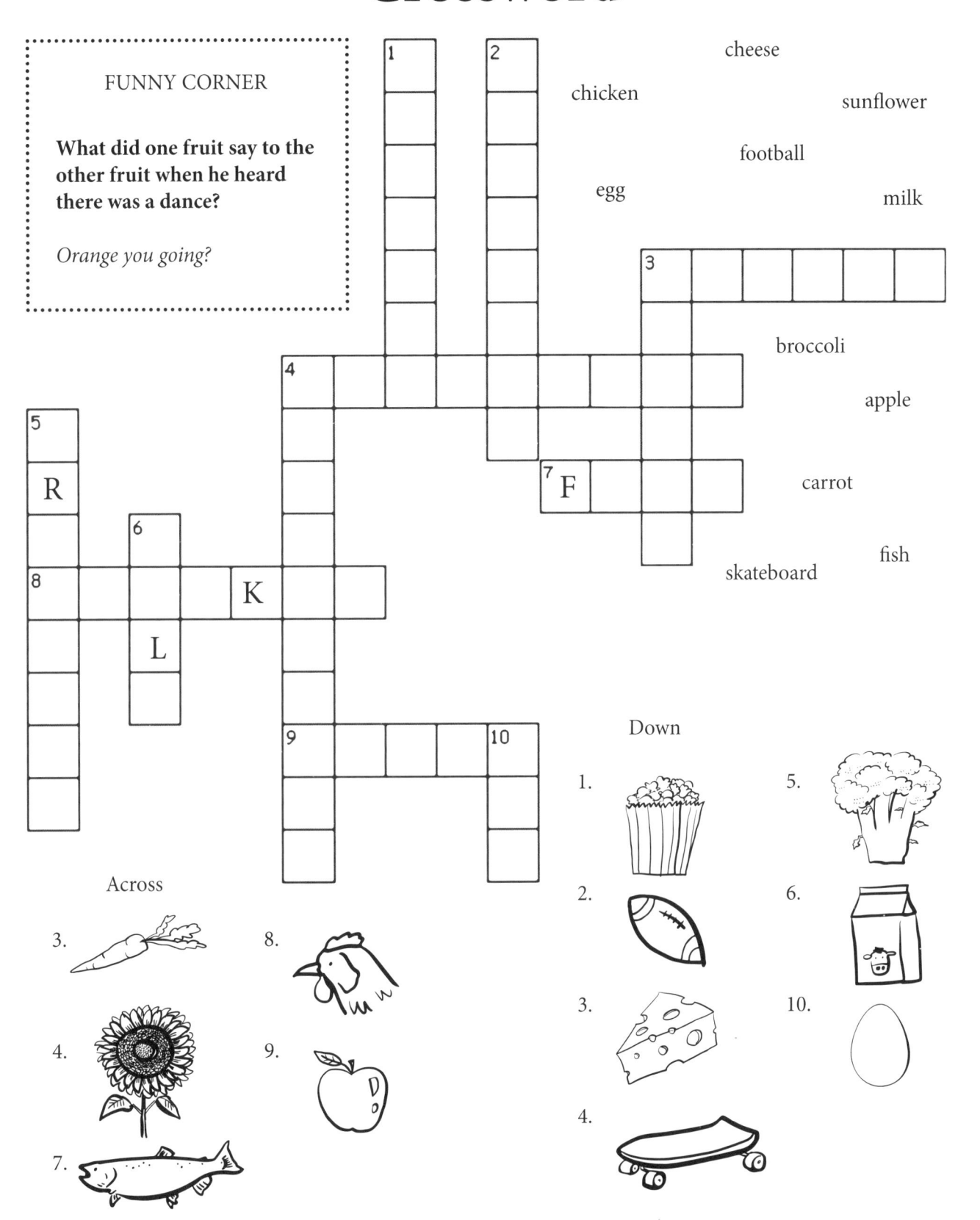

FUNNY CORNER

What did one fruit say to the other fruit when he heard there was a dance?

Orange you going?

cheese
chicken
sunflower
football
egg
milk
broccoli
apple
carrot
fish
skateboard

Across

3. (carrot)
4. (sunflower)
7. (fish)
8. (chicken)
9. (apple)

Down

1. (popcorn)
2. (football)
3. (cheese)
4. (skateboard)
5. (broccoli)
6. (milk)
10. (egg)

Healthy Habits text by Floyd Stokes. Illustrations © Sheena Hisiro.

Healthy Eating

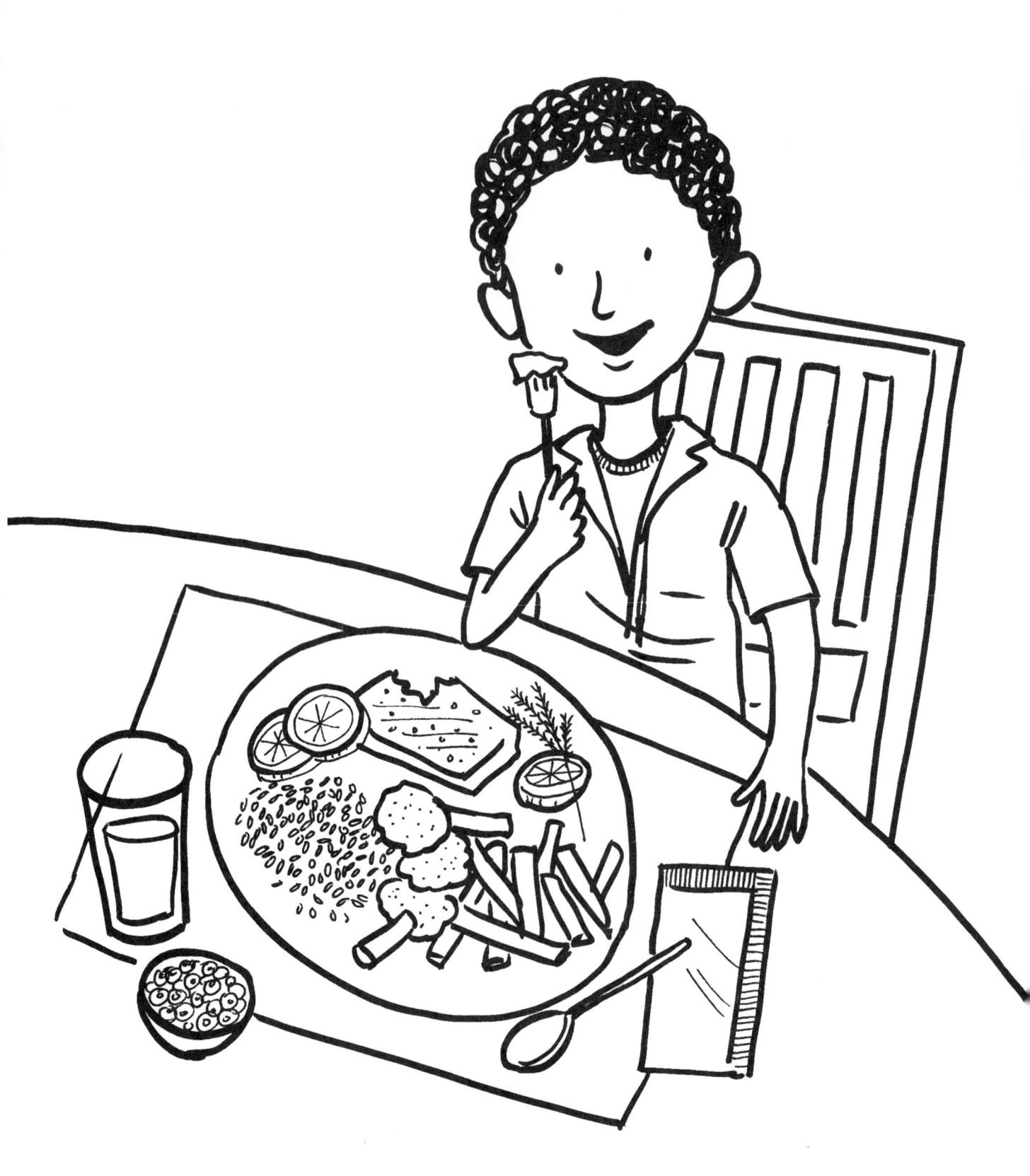

Spot the Difference Answers

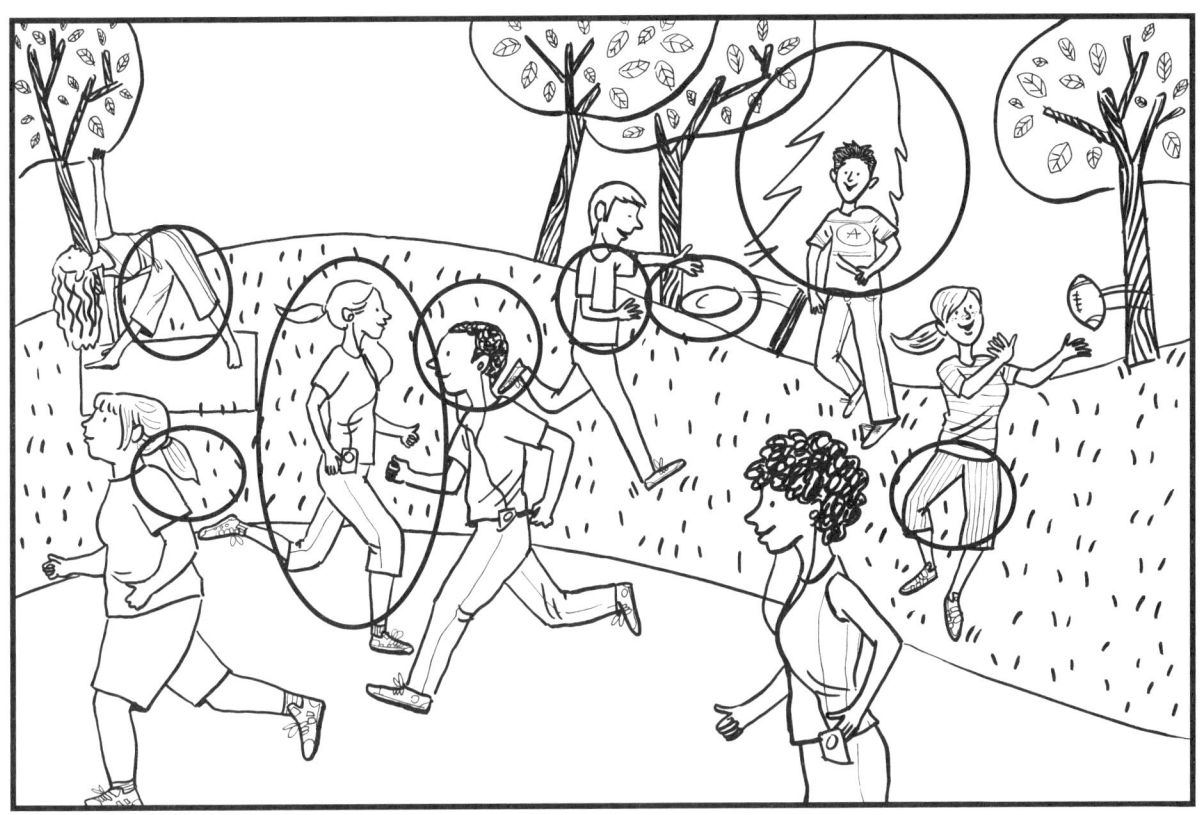

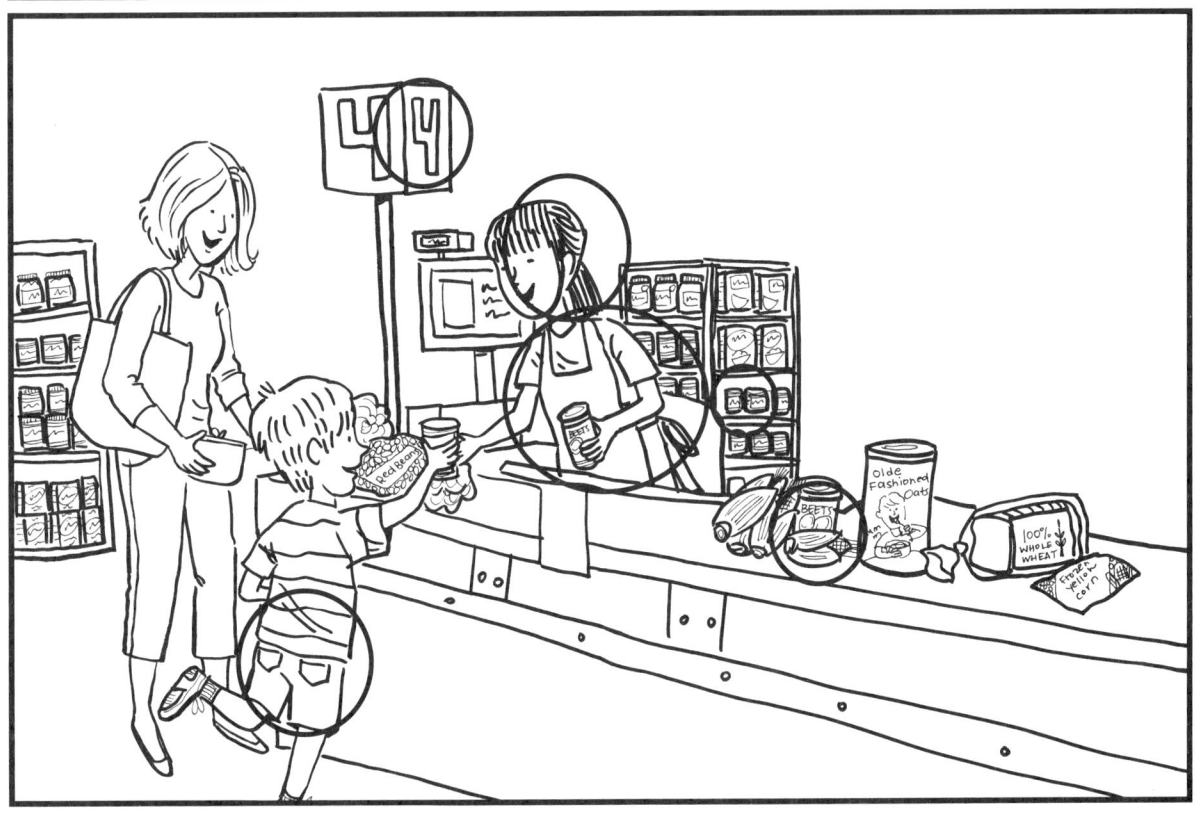

Healthy Habits text by Floyd Stokes. Illustrations © Sheena Hisiro.

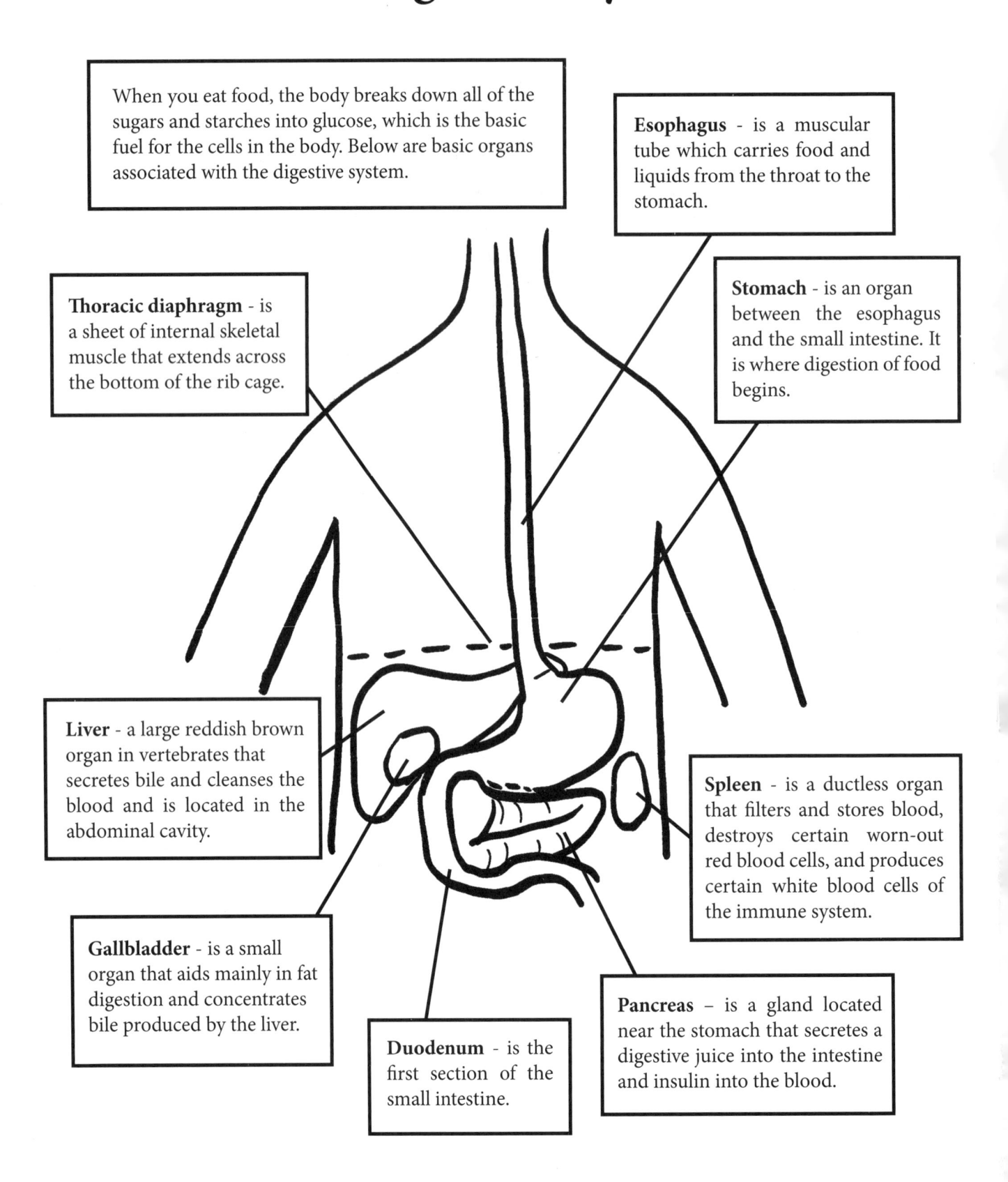

The Digestive System

When you eat food, the body breaks down all of the sugars and starches into glucose, which is the basic fuel for the cells in the body. Below are basic organs associated with the digestive system.

Esophagus - is a muscular tube which carries food and liquids from the throat to the stomach.

Thoracic diaphragm - is a sheet of internal skeletal muscle that extends across the bottom of the rib cage.

Stomach - is an organ between the esophagus and the small intestine. It is where digestion of food begins.

Liver - a large reddish brown organ in vertebrates that secretes bile and cleanses the blood and is located in the abdominal cavity.

Spleen - is a ductless organ that filters and stores blood, destroys certain worn-out red blood cells, and produces certain white blood cells of the immune system.

Gallbladder - is a small organ that aids mainly in fat digestion and concentrates bile produced by the liver.

Duodenum - is the first section of the small intestine.

Pancreas – is a gland located near the stomach that secretes a digestive juice into the intestine and insulin into the blood.

Healthy Habits text by Floyd Stokes. Illustrations © Sheena Hisiro.